POSITIVE
Psychology Approaches
to DEMENTIA

of related interest

Living Better with Dementia
Good Practice and Innovation for the Future
Shibley Rahman
Forewords by Kate Swaffer, Chris Roberts and Beth Britton
ISBN 978 1 84905 600 7
eISBN 978 1 78450 062 7

Doll Therapy in Dementia Care
Evidence and Practice
Gary Mitchell
ISBN 978 1 84905 570 3
eISBN 978 1 78450 007 8

Dementia, Culture and Ethnicity
Issues for All
Edited by Julia Botsford and Karen Harrison Dening
Foreword by Alistair Burns
ISBN 978 1 84905 486 7
eISBN 978 0 85700 881 7

How We Think About Dementia
Personhood, Rights, Ethics, the Arts and What They Mean for Care
Julian C. Hughes
ISBN 978 1 84905 477 5
eISBN 978 0 85700 855 8

POSITIVE
Psychology Approaches
to DEMENTIA

Edited *by* CHRIS CLARKE
and EMMA WOLVERSON

Foreword by Christine Bryden

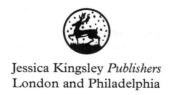

Jessica Kingsley *Publishers*
London and Philadelphia

The epigraph on page 133 is reproduced with kind permission from the author.
The epigraph on page 213 is reproduced from Baldwin and Capstick
with kind permission from McGraw-Hill Education.

First published in 2016
by Jessica Kingsley Publishers
73 Collier Street
London N1 9BE, UK
and
400 Market Street, Suite 400
Philadelphia, PA 19106, USA

www.jkp.com

Copyright © Jessica Kingsley Publishers 2016
Foreword copyright © Christine Bryden 2016

Front cover image source: rgbstock.com.

Library of Congress Cataloging in Publication Data
Names: Clarke, Chris (Psychologist), editor. | Wolverson, Emma, editor.
Title: Positive psychology approaches to dementia / edited by Chris Clarke
    and Emma Wolverson ; foreword by Christine Bryden.
Description: London ; Philadelphia : Jessica Kingsley Publishers, [2016] |
    Includes bibliographical references and index.
Identifiers: LCCN 2016012777 | ISBN 9781849056106 (alk. paper)
Subjects: LCSH: Dementia--Patients--Care. | Positive psychology. |
    Dementia--Treatment.
Classification: LCC RC521 .P667 2016 | DDC 616.8/3--dc23 LC record
available at https://urldefense.proofpoint.com/v2/url?u=https-3A__lccn.
loc.gov_2016012777&d=BQIFAg&c=euGZstcaTDllvimEN8b7jXrwqOf-
v5A_CdpgnVfiiMM&r=4EemtO9R1x-uacXap7EaQ1RHPq9-MnYBwnfuC-
ulpHU&m=BQArmhgv2XY-opm2CUT2pLdcwrXxEC5bknofrM1-5cs&
s=35ydryyySdIwvEZxC1zq69vTQHqNerebYMMt60f4b8w&e=

British Library Cataloguing in Publication Data
A CIP catalogue record for this book is available from the British Library

ISBN 978 1 84905 610 6
eISBN 978 1 78450 077 1

Printed and bound in the United States

CONTENTS

FOREWORD

I have lived well with dementia now for over 20 years, and in that time have seen a gradual move away from the negative narratives that have excluded the voices of those of us with the lived experience. This new work, edited by Chris Clarke and Emma Wolverson, now bursts onto the scene with compassion and understanding for hearing our voice to uncover what truly gives us a sense of well-being in life.

If only this work, this type of thinking, had been available when I was first diagnosed, how different my experience would have been! It has been a struggle to be heard, in the face of disbelief that I could speak, let alone find meaning and purpose in life. There is great promise for an even more positive social discourse of living well with dementia, and this work makes an extremely important contribution. Each step on that journey after diagnosis can be enriched by positive psychology so as to maximise our well-being. We can move on from living in dementia-friendly communities, towards being enriched by living in dementia-positive communities, which support us to find meaning and self-realisation in our lives.

The editors have brought together a critical overview of the current state of theoretical and empirical research in regard to the potential of positive psychology for enhancing the eudemonic well-being of people with dementia. In so doing, they have carefully identified gaps and proposed a strong rationale for exciting ways forward in developing a sound framework for positive psychology for all of us living well with dementia, as well as for our caregivers.

The chapters in this valuable resource focus on positive outcomes, countering the dominant biomedical discourse of negativity and loss, which has led to the stigma and fear that surround dementia. Instead of attempting solely to minimise medical so-called 'symptoms' of dementia, such as depression and anxiety, psycho-social interventions offer great promise of enhancing positive experiences.

In examining research to date, both qualitative as well as quantitative, the editors identify a need for further work based in sound theoretical frameworks. These would underpin research into the aspects of personal qualities, social environment and psycho-social process. What exactly is needed for us to flourish and grow, demonstrating resilience in the face of our dementia diagnosis? How can our well-being be measured, predicted, sustained and encouraged?

I found it reassuring to note that there was a balanced and nuanced view, which cautioned against ignoring negativity or apportioning blame to those of us who cannot rise above or through our experience of dementia. This balance is seen in the clear discussion of how well-being might result from the interplay between positive and negative aspects of our lives, with resilience and growth being able to result even from negative experiences.

There is a systematic exploration of research on the positive experiences and attributes that underlie personhood in dementia. Work is reviewed that examines the issues of interdependence and reciprocity in relationships, and the need for relationship-centred care, which support both those of us with dementia, as well as our caregivers, to discover a sense of well-being. Again there is a welcome counter-narrative to such language as 'burden' and 'stress', towards discovering positive aspects of caregiving.

This seminal work is a sound and thorough analysis of the current understanding of positive psychology and its potential in dementia. It re-balances the narrative towards living well with dementia, as attested to by many of us who are experts in the lived experience. Most importantly, it is a signpost to further work in the quest to enhance our ability to live well with dementia, with the help of positive psychology.

Positive psychology could and should be at the forefront of the development of dementia policy, programmes and services. Paramount is the need to listen to our lived experience and to focus on what really matters to those of us doing our best to live well with dementia, while balancing our positive and negative experiences regardless of the stigma and fear we face in today's society. Despite living with dementia, we can find meaning, such as in embodied moments of flow, creativity, humour, spirituality and connectedness – even of wisdom, growth and transcendence. There is a sense of moving forward and living in the now.

This book teaches us what it means to be human and to live a life of meaning and purpose, despite, through and with dementia. Positive psychology is a seismic shift in seeing us with new eyes – the world has truly shifted on its axis since my diagnosis all those years ago! We are moving away from the biomedical view of loss, symptoms and pathology, away from our negative stereotyping as sufferers or victims. Now we can stand tall as survivors with the hope of a meaningful, purposeful life in which we can find well-being, supported by positive psychology.

The clarity of the arguments offered in this book and the way it clearly signposts to a future of positivity and living well with dementia have given me great optimism for all those being diagnosed with dementia today and into the future. There are new horizons opening up of well-being, growth and transformation. We can find meaning in the chaos of life, and so inspire others as we flourish and live well with dementia.

Having lived through the transformation of a life interrupted by a diagnosis of dementia, I find inspiration in positive psychology. It offers the promise of helping us and our caregivers to find a helpful balance between positivity and negativity, towards a life of well-being, coping with resilience with the reality of decline and death.

I am daring to hope, daring to believe, in a society that no longer excludes, fears and stigmatises all of us who are living well with dementia.

Christine Bryden
March 2016
www.christinebryden.com
Author of *Who Will I Be When I Die?*,
Dancing with Dementia,
Nothing About Us, Without Us,
(Jessica Kingsley Publishers) and
Before I Forget
(Penguin Australia)

ACKNOWLEDGEMENTS

Our contributors have provided truly outstanding and inspiring chapters that each deserve recognition in their own right. The creation of this book depended on their generous and thoughtful efforts.

Various family members, friends and colleagues, including my esteemed co-editor, have helped sustain my commitment to this book and the vision that underpins it. I am deeply grateful to each of them.

This book was inspired by the lived experiences of people with dementia. I drew inspiration from a particular individual: Harold Walter 'Nobby' Clarke, a creative, playful, generous and persevering gentleman who lived with dementia.

Chris Clarke

I'm fortunate enough to have been mentored by some truly inspirational practitioners who've taught me to see strengths and possibilities everywhere. Amongst them, I'd especially like to say thank you to Esme, Peter, Janet and Karen.

I'd also like to thank my wonderful family – particularly Eddy, Charlotte Rose, and our new addition, who bring so much love, humour, hope and joy to my life.

In memory of Eileen – a remarkable woman.

Emma Wolverson

We jointly extend our gratitude and respect to members of the 'Butterflies Memory-loss Support Group' (coordinated by June Cooke; see www.butterflies.org.uk) who, with amazing enthusiasm and perceptiveness, created themed artworks to complement the majority of the chapters of this book. We further thank Tricia Boulton at www.facetphotography.co.uk for kindly bringing her expertise to bear on creating beautiful images of these artworks.

INTRODUCTION

It would be typical to begin a book on dementia by describing the plethora of problems and burdens that it can impose on individuals, healthcare systems and society. As readers will be aware, across the globe increasing numbers of us are encountering dementia as we age and, as we do, we may face significant challenges to our well-being, our sense of identity and the continuity of our close relationships. Policy makers and providers of health and social care increasingly have to respond strategically to dementia as a public health priority as well as a significant social and economic pressure.

However, to begin this book with a negative and *problematising* narrative about dementia would be at odds with its central aim, which is to explore the psychological states and experiences that might make it possible not merely to *live with* the condition but to *live positively*. Although dementia remains a stigmatised and feared condition that is easily described in terms of loss, decline and pathology, this book instead seeks to explore an alternative, positive narrative that reflects people's actual experiences of living with dementia.

Why create a book that attempts to explore these issues and promote such a narrative? It is easy to be sceptical of the notion of maintaining well-being and having positive personal and social experiences whilst living with dementia. It may be easy to assume, as many previously have done, that the changes in cognitive, social and functional abilities that occur in dementia severely limit if not preclude genuine experiences of well-being. A natural concern might also be that in directing attention towards the possibility of such experiences we risk invalidating people's negative experiences and struggles.

We cannot ignore or underestimate these possibilities. However, to consider the possibility of living positively with dementia we must recognise the influence of biomedical discourses of loss and pathology that usually surround the condition. Such discourses imply that dementia automatically dominates and devastates a person's everyday life. As such, people living with dementia are seldom asked if (and how) they still experience achievement, enjoyment, love, hope, humour, growth and spirituality. The assumption that people with dementia do not and cannot have these kinds of experiences is therefore maintained.

Whether living with dementia, at a subjective level, involves the degree of suffering that might be assumed is actually far from clear and, in recent years, accounts of positive experiences in living with dementia have emerged. This has coincided with a timely re-appraisal of the value of open inquiry into people's lived experiences, based on phenomenological and constructionist perspectives and qualitative research methods. At the same time, principles and constructs from the field of positive psychology are increasingly being applied to understanding how people age successfully and can respond positively to adversity related to living with long-term health conditions. So-called *second wave* positive psychology approaches are very relevant here as they are concerned with how positive and negative states interact and are contextually defined.

Documenting and understanding such processes and experiences in dementia have important implications in terms of enhancing conceptual accounts of well-being and quality of life, as well as re-contextualising and de-stigmatising the condition.

Since the majority of people who encounter dementia do so in late life, a key feature of this book is how positive experiences occur in the context of ageing as well as in relation to dementia-related changes and challenges. We hope that the book will not be considered irrelevant to people attempting to live well with young-onset dementia, but we also recognise that this involves its own particular themes and challenges, which deserve attention in their own right.

Chapters 1 and 2 of this book together introduce the background and rationale for a contextualised, positive psychology-informed approach to fully understanding people's positive lived experiences in living with dementia in later life. In Chapter 1, Elspeth Stirling introduces positive psychology, its central principles and key models. She sets the scene for subsequent chapters by orientating the reader to aspects of the positive psychology of ageing, such as positive developmental changes in personality and emotion regulation, and by highlighting how positive states and experiences, such as resilience and optimism, can shape adjustment and well-being in chronic illness. This serves as an important prelude to the rest of the book by indicating how we might frame living with dementia as akin to living well with a chronic health condition in the context of ageing.

In Chapter 2, in collaboration with Esme Moniz-Cook, we describe the background to a positive, person-centred approach to understanding well-being in dementia. In support, we present the findings of a systematic literature review of positive lived experiences in dementia and consider how a contextualised, positive, person-centred approach potentially offers an alternative frame for negative discourses that traditionally surround the condition.

Subsequent chapters each address separate positive psychology constructs or themes and their potential application to understanding living well with dementia. Each chapter is accompanied and illustrated by an image of creative work undertaken by the *Butterflies* dementia support and advocacy group, based in Kingston-upon-Hull, UK. Each creative piece represents the theme of the chapter.

In Chapter 3, Alison Phinney discusses the important concepts of well-being and quality of life in relation to dementia, highlighting, in particular, how aspects of the former may not always be fully captured when we attempt to assess the latter. In Chapters 4 and 5, we describe the ways in which hope and humour, respectively, might contribute to well-being in dementia and illustrate how personal experiences of these constructs in dementia can have varying meanings and significance. In Chapter 6, Phyllis Braudy Harris explores resilience and how this overarching concept offers an alternative to narrow models of successful ageing, therefore promoting a more inclusive approach to understanding how people with dementia can continue to use personal and social assets to maintain well-being in the face of the varied challenges the condition brings.

Chapter 7, by Kirsty Patterson and Emma Wolverson, centres on a challenging question: whether the personal growth known to be possible in ageing and in relation to adversity due to ill-health or trauma might also be possible for people living with dementia. In doing so, this chapter examines the potentially controversial possibility that some people may experience personally transformative experiences *because of* dementia, which, in turn, lead to the experience of new and different forms of well-being. Chapters 8 and 9 cover the important constructs of creativity (John Killick) and spirituality and wisdom (Andrew Norris and Bob Woods). In doing so, these contributors explore how experiences in each of these domains are not only possible in dementia but are potentially pivotal in preserving identity, personhood and well-being.

Chapters 10 and 11 extend the focus of the book by examining how positive psychology might be applied to relationships in dementia caregiving and to understanding positive experiences of caregiving. In exploring how a 'Senses Framework' can be applied to enriched, relational caregiving in dementia, Tony Ryan and Mike Nolan illustrate in Chapter 10 how the well-being of the person with dementia is inextricably linked with the psychological health not only of family carers and staff but also of whole organisations. Catherine Quinn highlights in Chapter 11 how positive aspects of caregiving can include individual experiences of meaning making, connectedness and growth, which may, in turn, be connected to the quality of care that family carers feel able to provide.

The list of constructs and issues addressed by this book is by no means exhaustive. In several ways this is an emerging field of study and, as we call for in Chapter 12, considerable further research is needed to explore how different aspects of positive well-being in dementia are experienced and best facilitated. In that final chapter we tentatively propose an initial meta-level framework for conceptualising positive experiences and outcomes in dementia and discuss some of the clinical and public policy implications of taking a contextualised, positive psychology approach to well-being in dementia.

Our own experiences of creating and editing this book and of conducting research into positive experiences in dementia reflect the *dialectics* of positive experiences and emotions. On the one hand, we have been inspired by how re-defining challenges and losses involved in dementia can be accompanied by, or even spur, experiences of hope, humour, resilience, meaning and connectedness, as people strive to maintain their well-being. On the other hand, there is the continuous need to bear in mind that not everyone living with dementia has such positive experiences. Expecting people with dementia to have these experiences would be invalidating and likely to promote further negative experiences.

Whilst we and our contributors deliberately pursue a positive 'counter-narrative' about dementia in this book, it would also be wrong to reduce the lived experience of dementia to any kind of dichotomous rhetoric. The reality of everybody's lives is, of course, far more complex; an interplay exists between our positive and negative emotions and experiences, which are defined subjectively and contextually and we believe this is perhaps more true for people living with dementia.

At the same time, this book intentionally draws attention to and celebrates everyday sources of wonder in the lives of people with dementia, as a reaction to nihilistic and othering discourses, which can effectively obscure the full nature of people's experiences. As Jon McGregor highlights in his novel *If Nobody Speaks of Remarkable Things* (2002), '...there are remarkable things all the time, right in front of us, but our eyes have like the clouds over the sun and our lives are paler and poorer if we do not see them for what they are. If nobody speaks of remarkable things, how can they be called remarkable?' (p.239).[1]

At its heart, this book speaks about how people with dementia can still experience and achieve 'remarkable things', not only in spite of but also because of dementia.

Chris Clarke and Emma Wolverson
July 2016

---

1   McGregor, J. (2002) *If Nobody Speaks of Remarkable Things*. London: Bloomsbury

Chapter 1

AGEING, HEALTH AND POSITIVE PSYCHOLOGY

Elspeth Stirling

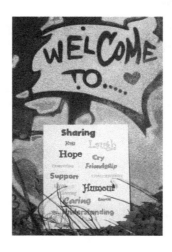

From the wall we sit on in earlier life, we see life through our filters of the time – unable to see beyond the veil into later life and condescendingly presuming that there is nothing but loss of what we value now. From the wall we sit on in later life, we have a very different vista. We experience emancipation, transcendence, connection and transformation in the new landscape opening out before us. We encounter challenges, unlike any experienced before, and are enriched with experiences of reciprocity, trust, humility, clarity, and urgency.

Elspeth Stirling

INTRODUCTION

Living into later life has become the normative experience in recent decades, at least in those parts of the world called 'developed' (Rosling, 2013). At the same time, happiness is increasingly considered a measure of social progress and a goal for public policy (Helliwell, Layard and Sachs, 2015). Whilst not universal, experiences of *living well* into later life, sustaining meaning and well-being despite the raised likelihood of experiencing transformational life challenges, are increasingly being reported (e.g. see Kok *et al.*, 2015). As a group, older people tend to exhibit more effective emotional regulation as well as increased well-being and life satisfaction in comparison with younger adults. As the possibility of ageing well has increasingly been acknowledged and promoted, public perceptions of later life are not as often overshadowed by negative or static stereotypes.

The rapidly diversifying field of positive psychology offers perspectives, conceptual models and empirical findings that are highly relevant to understanding how people might live well as they age and encounter health problems of different kinds. The potential application of PP to furthering our understanding of how people age well in spite of objective adversity such as illness is therefore the core focus of this chapter. Influential PP perspectives and models and their conceptual roots are described and the chapter examines how these might help to progress our understanding of psychological development and the improvement of well-being in relation to ageing and to health. PP is highly relevant to extending our understanding of the experience of meaning and value in later life and in illness. The perspective can therefore contribute significantly to the development of psycho-social interventions aimed at maintaining and improving well-being in the context of age-related physical and psychological challenges.

INTRODUCING POSITIVE PSYCHOLOGY

Clinicians and researchers working with people in all parts of the life-span recognised some decades ago the need for a new paradigm within science to move away from the shackles of illness-based and pathology-focused accounts of human experience and distress. Positive psychology (PP) is the field of science that is devoted to the study and theory of positive functioning and well-being across individual, interpersonal, organisational and societal domains (Rusk and Waters, 2014).

Seligman (1999) is widely regarded as initiating the field of PP as an antithesis to the historical dominance of pathology and negativity in mainstream psychology. PP is therefore deliberately concerned with human strengths and virtues, positive subjective experiences, the nature and measurement of well-being and, increasingly, the social and environmental conditions that facilitate positive experiences and well-being. PP carries the basic assumption that human beings are intrinsically motivated to develop their psychological strengths, seek positive emotions and achieve meaning through their activities, experiences and social connections across the life-span.

PP is a non-pathologising approach. Human distress is on a continuum with normal experiences and linked to how able social and physical environments are to provide people with opportunities to use their strengths and have authentic optimal experiences. At the same time, recent PP perspectives (e.g. see Wong, 2011) open up the possibility that positive and negative experiences and states can co-occur and interact, a position highly relevant to understanding well-being in adversity and illness (e.g. see Aspinwall and Tedeschi, 2010). A key driver in the continued development of the applied PP movement has been the need to understand the processes that occur naturally when positive functioning follows in the aftermath of adverse circumstances (Seligman, 2005) with the purpose of applying this knowledge to helping people achieve optimal, or 'beyond baseline', outcomes even in the face of adversity (Keyes and Lopez, 2005).

PP is not about making people think positively. Most people will have come across populist, mandating 'think positive' mantras that purport to be passports to good health, relationships and success. Serious concerns about this so-called 'tyranny of the positives' include that it involves the suppression of negative emotions and experiences, and the denial of real suffering, as well as an intimidating promotion of false hope and victim-blaming (Aspinwall and Tedeschi, 2010). Instead, modern PP perspectives (e.g. see Lomas and Ivtzan, 2015) acknowledge and work with a dialectic, or dynamic interplay, between positive and negative psychological processes and outcomes, and seek to shed light on how individuals might attempt to find ways to flourish even in the context of changes and challenges encountered over the life-span. To flourish is to live well and achieve an optimal level of functioning characterised by positive emotions, positive relationships, mastery, growth and resilience (see Fredrickson and Losada, 2005). However, the notion of flourishing is not context-free and does not have to mean a naïve denial of negative experiences and emotions. By implication, to ask the question of what enables people to flourish necessitates a fully conscious understanding of the context and impact of suffering and the processes underlying adaptive functioning in the face of adversity. Our understanding of the experiences and processes (both the positive and, potentially, the negative) that foster well-being therefore requires a contextualised approach.

There are various levels to the contexts within which people might find ways to flourish in spite of the experience of adversity. Personal and social contexts may include factors such as coping style, personality, cognitive ability, life stage, quality of interpersonal relationships, perceived social support, socio-economic status and more. In their interaction, such factors influence the capacity we have to maintain and improve well-being as we age. Furthermore, as Lomas (2016) describes, personal and social contexts shape the meaning of our experiences to the extent that what in one context (temporal or spatial) may appear negative (e.g. trauma), in another can be, or can become, positive (e.g. transformational growth).

The social context of well-being is an area that has been relatively neglected in the PP literature to date. Yet it would be difficult to overstate the importance that our relationships and our connections with communities and society each have in shaping and fostering our capacity to flourish. An influential perspective in this regard is social role valorisation (SRV), which focuses on how life sharing with valued community members is likely to enhance positive subjective experiences and provide more opportunities for developing positive competencies. By developing valued social roles that are supported by communities, marginalised people can be afforded protection from a 'vicious circle' of impairment and internalised stigma. SRV has for a long time appealed to a wide range of human service providers for the reason that it offers a robust theory that has no place for either victim-blaming or denial of suffering (Flynn and Lemay, 1999; Wolfensberger, 2000). What has been less obvious is that SRV and PP are closely allied in their shared focus on understanding the complex person–environment processes that underlie positive experiences and competencies. Both perspectives approach this by studying how people flourish naturally, while SRV particularly emphasises the powerful role of being valued within the mainstream of society for the promotion of well-being and for protection in a time of crisis or marginalisation. PP as a field also exists in a social context of ethics and values where conflicting views can predominate, particularly about contentious issues in later life, such as the provision and funding of care, the marginalisation of older people and the right to die. It is helpful to clarify that PP, as an empirical approach, does not necessarily purport to answer ethical or values questions. These are ultimately answered by society, not by science. Values questions typically ask: 'Is that event considered *desirable*, widely, for valued people in that society?' Ethics questions typically ask: 'Is that event considered *acceptable*, generally, in that society?' In contrast, empirical questions typically ask: 'Is that event (or process) *effective* in relation to the person achieving the designated outcome?' PP has typically been concerned with the latter category of question in terms of how factors such as hope, resilience and altruism contribute to positive well-being outcomes for individuals, groups and societies (Linley and Joseph, 2004). Despite this, it should be openly acknowledged that PP perspectives carry an inherent value position; at individual through to social levels of application, positive well-being, optimal experiences, and personal and civic virtues are all held to be personally and socially valuable. Thus, PP is not a value-free perspective but neither is it prescriptive in relation to how people should pursue well-being and find meaning in their lives (Linley and Joseph, 2004).

A contextualised approach to applying PP must also take into account the environmental context within which personal and collective human well-being is experienced. At the time of writing, crises are occurring in the social and physical environment; individuals and organisations across the globe will increasingly be called upon to adapt their habitual behaviours radically and positively. The future security of all life depends on the human capacity to embrace, adapt to and optimise changing world conditions including climate change, global warming, resource-depletion, population growth, mass-migration and social inequalities. At this level, human happiness, socio-political stability and the ecological well-being of the planet can all be seen as inter-linked, as noted by Helliwell, Layard and Sachs (2015, p.5):

> The concepts of happiness and well-being are very likely to help guide progress towards sustainable development. [...]

[UN Sustainable Development Goals (SDGs)] are designed to help countries to achieve economic, social and environmental objectives in harmony, thereby leading to higher levels of well-being for the present and future generations.

PP has much to offer in terms of understanding how human flourishing develops in environmental adversity. We now have statistical data spanning 50 years that shows that populations increasingly value aspirational goals related to social well-being and happiness (Rosling, 2013). Specifically, healthy life expectancy, perceived social support, trust, generosity, freedom to make life decisions, fairness and the environment are identified as crucial to personal well-being. Interestingly, income is relevant but not of highest importance. Humans experience increased well-being it seems when they feel part of a meaningful whole for which they share responsibility. These are the important underpinnings for happiness and coping well when adverse circumstances come along.

KEY POSITIVE PSYCHOLOGY MODELS AND FRAMEWORKS

In recent years, notable attempts have been made to provide overarching conceptualisations of positive states and experiences and how these are achieved and maintained. It is useful to outline three of these models in order to further explore how a PP perspective can be brought to develop our understanding of well-being in ageing and in relation to health.

VALUES IN ACTION (VIA)

Proposed by Peterson and Seligman (2004), this framework comprises 24 character strengths, or positive personal traits, that are categorised into six sets of virtues – morally valued dispositions that apply across cultures. Virtues span wisdom and knowledge (including creativity and curiosity), courage (which includes perseverance and zest), humanity (including love and kindness), justice (e.g. fairness and also teamwork), temperance (which includes forgiveness) and transcendence, which involves character strengths such as humour, hope and gratitude, held to 'forge connections to the larger universe and provide meaning'

(Peterson and Park, 2009, p.27). Character strengths and virtues, in this approach, make possible positive subjective experiences and flourishing, and evidence supports a strong association between life-satisfaction, well-being and particular strengths of character, including love, hope, gratitude, curiosity and zest (see Peterson and Park, 2009). The VIA framework can also frame goals for interventions (i.e. building and cultivating strengths), conceptualised as individual internal resources. In addition, there is some evidence that character strengths emerge from adversity and loss (e.g. see Schueller *et al.*, 2014), reflecting the value of a dialectical understanding of positive experiences. If misunderstood, however, this approach could result in blaming the individual who has not developed a particular character strength after experiencing adversity.

POSITIVE EMOTION, ENGAGEMENT, RELATIONSHIPS, MEANING, ACCOMPLISHMENT (PERMA)

Proposed by Seligman and colleagues (see Seligman, 2011), this framework identifies five measureable dimensions of well-being – positive emotion, engagement with activity (flow), positive relationships, meaning (a sense of purpose and a connection with something greater than oneself) and accomplishment. These are primarily framed as positive outcomes, which in combination define a state of flourishing. Empirical work supports this multi-dimensional approach to defining well-being and indicates that these are separable dimensions (e.g. see Kern *et al.*, 2015). This approach has the advantage of combining social factors and relationships with individual internal resources in defining positive well-being, and it provides an overarching framework for the measurement of well-being and flourishing. However, if misunderstood or seen out of context, the model could be perceived as a 'mindless mantra' towards achieving happiness.

FIVE DOMAINS OF POSITIVE FUNCTIONING (DPF-5)

Proposed by Rusk and Waters in 2014, this model represents a system-based approach to understanding the processes that underpin positive psycho-social functioning. The model was empirically derived from a cluster analysis carried out on terms used in a wide range of published documents concerning PP. The emerging clusters were interpreted as referring to how individuals function to achieve well-being. These are:

- *attention and awareness* to positive aspects of information – this relates also to mindfulness

- *comprehension and coping* with adversity arising from the prediction of future possibilities – this relates to important constructs such as expectancy, hope, post-traumatic growth and resilience

- *emotions* applied to understanding what is in the environment

- *goals and habits* selectively influenced by individual values

- *virtues and relationships*, which influence individual pro-social behaviour, altruism, gratitude, empathy and forgiveness.

The domains described in this model together constitute a complex, dynamic system in which each domain interacts with and influences the others – a conceptualisation consistent with the available evidence regarding positive experiences and positive functioning. For example, positive emotions can broaden attention, and the prediction of future possibilities can increase flexible action and enhance relationships. In this system, mutually reinforcing positive interactions between domains take place, resulting in 'upward spirals' of general positive well-being (Frederickson, 2004). Whilst it is a broad and highly conceptual framework, the DPF-5 does provide important empirically driven insights into the processes that underlie personal growth, well-being and positive subjective experiences, and how people might vary in these experiences.

POSITIVE PSYCHOLOGY IN LATER LIFE

There is a particularly strong effect of age stereotyping in older 'developed' societies. People in later life are dealt with in ways that have long been unacceptable for other groups. Such societies use technology to pursue the creation of 'the perfect individual' and 'eternal life'. In this context, ageing is seen as the 'breakdown of the machine' and there is an implied failure of a technical fix. This, it can be argued, sustains a denial of death and perpetuates unconscious, defensive eugenic measures (concealment) and exit-making for frail people in later life (Smith, 2003; Sudnow, 1967). As a result, fear has been possibly the most common feeling associated with the concept of ageing in such societies. However, this is not a pattern replicated world-wide. Crucially, when we ask about people's actual lived experience and scientifically examine positive experiences and coping, then we uncover contradictory evidence – of a reality that development in later life can bring a beneficial clarity of values and an enjoyable landscape of experiences and competencies.

It has been known for some time that, contrary to popular assumptions, most people have a positive experience of later life (Diener and Suh, 1998; Williamson, 2005) and there is now mounting evidence that several measurable positive factors increase in later life – namely well-being, emotional regulation and life satisfaction (Tornstam, 2011; Urry and Gross, 2010). Moreover, the clearest connections between happiness and the possible processes that underlie happiness are found in people in later life (perceived social support, trust, generosity, freedom to make life decisions), suggesting the possibility that for science the study of later life may offer the clearest view of how well-being is attained and maintained.

The concept of successful ageing – maintaining objective and subjective physical and psychological health in late life – has been recognised for some time but is also subject to debate (see Cosco *et al.*, 2014 for a review of the ways successful ageing has been defined). A key issue is whether successful ageing is truly meaningful if only defined in terms of maintaining an objective level of positive physical health and functioning. In contrast, positive ageing is described by Vaillant (2004) as relating to indices of objective physical and mental health status combined with subjective perceptions of health and life satisfaction. As thinking about well-being in ageing has progressed, the focus has shifted away from minimising losses and maintaining objective health towards understanding the processes that might underpin subjective well-being, growth and transformational functioning in later life, even if objective health status is less than optimal. Worth (2016) highlights how developmental processes over the life-span (such as negotiating key psycho-social tasks) might add to a person's profile of personal strengths in later life and therefore contribute to positive changes in well-being in spite of age-related physical and psychological challenges. Being able to sustain love, engage in creative activities, transcend our immediate circumstances and find meaning are potentially key aspects of positive ageing that are facilitated by such life-span developmental processes. Positive, or 'mature', coping (e.g. the use of humour in the face of adversity) has also been seen as an aspect of positive ageing and is strongly linked with increased longevity and sustained health in later life (see Malone *et al.*, 2013).

EMOTION REGULATION AND LATER LIFE

Early observations of reduced fluctuation in emotions in later life have more recently been framed in terms of different strategies of *emotion regulation* (Urry and Gross, 2010). Generally speaking, older people tend to be better than younger people at regulating positive and negative emotion, but the processes underpinning this may be varied. The key age-related changes, and how they contribute to increased well-being, seem to involve the following:

- With greater age, people are better at predicting emotional arousal in situations and therefore can select situations better – avoiding unnecessary negative emotions and selecting situations where positive emotions are more likely.

- Attention is more selective to positive information in later life – making attentional deployment more likely to be productive of positive experiences.

- Emotional arousal is often associated with the re-appraisal that follows in the aftermath of choices; with greater age this activation effect is moderated by cognitive control with a consequent decrease in negative emotions.

Socio-emotional selectivity theory (Lockenhoff and Carstensen, 2004) offers a conceptual account of the motivational processes that might underpin improved emotional regulation in ageing. This theory posits that an awareness of time being finite (i.e. personal mortality) shifts a person's time perspective towards the present and leads to a re-prioritising of personal goals in favour of experiencing positive over negative emotion and maintaining close emotional bonds with significant others. In later life, emotionally meaningful goals and activities are therefore prioritised. These include:

- *generative activities* – for example, passing on one's knowledge, taking responsibility for future life and generations

- *present oriented goals* – for example, alleviating aversive symptoms or interacting with loved objects

- *reducing network size* – for example, choosing valued partners and opting out of peripheral social partners

- *focusing on stimuli with emotional valence* – for example, music, photographs, etc.

In summary, the regulation of emotion becomes stronger in later life, promoting improved moderation of negative emotion and more decisive decision making in crises. Increased socio-emotional selectivity can strengthen the motivation to experience positive emotions and seek satisfaction in valued relationships, and it promotes a growing experience of being part of the regenerative cycle of life.

GEROTRANSCENDENCE

Expectations about later life have historically been dominated by beliefs that ageing is about loss, misery, disengagement and regret, despite evidence to the contrary. The theory of gerotranscendence captures more accurately how individuals describe their own experiences of later life, as well as explaining research findings of high life satisfaction in ageing (Tornstam, 2011). The lived experience of later life is described as a developmental pattern typically involving increased life satisfaction, reduced self-occupation and a heightened sense of affinity with others across the boundaries of time and place, summed up as a sense of being part of the whole natural environment.

Gerotranscendence is seen to take place along three dimensions:

- In the *cosmic dimension*, the experience of time is redefined, such that the past and present can be experienced more as one, and one's own life is seen as part of a chain of events rather than as an isolated point in the universe.

- In *the dimension of self*, decreases in self-centredness allow the person to look more in an outward direction and develop a stronger sense of being an integral part of the whole of reality.

- In the *social dimension*, interest in superficial socialising and peripheral relationships is relaxed, making way for increased satisfaction with valued relationships and fostering the capacity for increased appreciation of a positive, contemplative solitude.

Tornstam (2011) estimates that high levels of gerotranscendence are reached naturally by around 20 per cent of older people. Emancipation from the roles and societal expectancies that predominate in mid-adult life is reported – for example, liberation from material, economic and production preoccupations, and increased tolerance of complexity in moral matters. The greatest barriers halting people's achievement of high transcendence in later life include the expectation many of us hold that later life will involve a continuation of the same values as in mid-adult life, as well as the imposition of erroneous interpretations by people in earlier life – for example, when they mistake the new joy in contemplation with 'depression' or 'slowing down'. These are examples of mid-life values imposed mistakenly on later life development. It seems likely that many people are stopped, or stop themselves, in the process of growing into later life by becoming trapped in these static expectancies.

CREATING AN ENVIRONMENT THAT PROMOTES WELL-BEING AND COPING IN LATER LIFE

The concept of thriving in late life has been used to describe an optimal state of living and well-being that depends on an interaction between a person, their social environment, and their physical environment (see Haight et al., 2002). This concept has significant implications for understanding how well-being is understood and improved for people living in certain kinds of environments, as it directs attention both to positive outcomes and the social contexts within which people strive to maintain well-being.

According to Bergland and Kirkevold (2006), the experience of thriving reflects 'an adjusted balance between the expectations of the individual and the capacity of the environment to accommodate the expectations' (p.689). On the one hand this involves a process of active adjustment of goals and expectations that is internal to the individual. Yet thriving is a reciprocal process and cannot occur in the absence of good quality care and social relationships, as experienced by the person in the context of a given setting.

More widely, thriving could therefore be said to relate to social contexts in which the most vulnerable endure the least threat to their position. Simultaneously, the life experiences of the more able members of society are enhanced by their understanding and appreciation not only of the unique needs of older people but, more importantly, their strengths in adversity.

These varied perspectives on well-being in ageing indicate how developmental processes across the life-span might interact with positive aspects of the social environment to foster and sustain positive emotions and experiences. As such, quality of life in ageing can hinge on congruence between assets and characteristics of the individual and the resources present in their environment. In turn, however, older people can play an active role in contributing to this transaction and contributing to the quality of life in their community (see Ranzijn, 2002).

The three factors below have been identified as important in creating an environment likely to promote well-being and the capacity for coping in later life, drawing on Lemay (1999) and Wolfensberger (1998):

- *Social roles relate to well-being.* There is evidence within psychology to demonstrate that having valued social roles in later life protects and enhances self-esteem, self-identity and serves as a buffer against adverse events (Cheston and Bender, 1999).

- *Members of a community are able to draw strength and resilience from the presence of its members who are closer to death/living with limiting conditions.* Opportunities to share life-defining experiences are likely to foster pro-social competencies and hope in community members of all ages. People in earlier life learn from seeing how their co-members of society in later life respond to adversities and cope naturally with significant life-defining difficulties. If people in later life are contained away from the mainstream of society, and/or are mainly talked about in terms of negative attributes (e.g. pity), then it is likely that the response to them will be fear and denial, leading to lost opportunities for learning resilience (see Stirling, 2010).

- *Disability and adversity are part of the natural range of experience in all life.* From our knowledge of the power of modelling in psychology, we know it is likely that the individual who witnesses how others in their community deal with life challenges will be more likely to develop adaptive behaviours themselves.

POSITIVE PSYCHOLOGY AND CHRONIC ILLNESS

Increasingly, empirical research demonstrates the value of positive traits, processes and experiences in relation to adjusting to, and living well with, chronic health conditions. Aspinwall and Tedeschi (2010) review evidence showing that factors such as optimism, benefit finding, positive affectivity and sense of coherence (to what degree people see life events as comprehensible, manageable and meaningful) can have both protective and ameliorating effects and help people adjust positively to long-term physical health conditions. Such positive factors may act beneficially on health via a number of inter-related pathways. For example, factors such as optimism and positive emotion may impact beneficially on the body's neurological, endocrine and immune systems but can also contribute to health through effects on coping, social support and greater adherence to rehabilitation programmes.

In addition to applications in health psychology, an early development in PP was a redefined understanding of mental health in relation to the notion of flourishing rather than pathology. Keyes and Lopez (2005) proposed a two-factor conceptualisation in which mental illness behaviours and psychological well-being can be viewed as separable (albeit linked) dimensions. Furthermore, in this framework, mental illness is related primarily to the absence of flourishing and of the conditions that might facilitate this. Psychological well-being goals can be pursued irrespective of where the person is on the continuum of mental illness symptoms; there is no condition that states that the person must 'get better' from mental illness before embarking towards psychological well-being goals (Wrzesniewski, 2005). Keyes and Lopez's (2005) analysis opens up new possibilities for the development of life skills that might enable people to live with, rather than be defined by, symptoms of a physical or mental illness. This approach has much in common with the modern concept of recovery in mental health.

Keyes' (2007) model of mental health focuses on the key subjective, psychological and social aspects of well-being. In later life, we may be equally as interested in the experience of chronic physical illness, given its varied forms, its association with ageing and the threat long-term conditions can pose to a person's well-being. Figure 1.1 outlines an adapted model based on that of Keyes (2007), with four possible *platforms* of coping skills, which relate to categories of well-being that may be experienced in relation to the real and perceived impact of physical health problems.

Psychological well-being

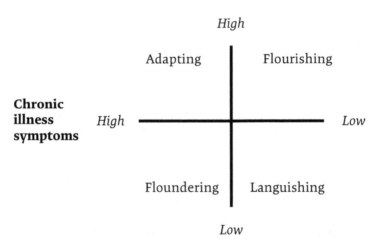

Figure 1.1: Applying the Keyes positive psychology model to chronic illness

A person might be said to be languishing where both psychological well-being and symptoms of a chronic health problem are low. That person may be vulnerable to a collapse of coping in the event of increased severity of chronic illness symptoms. Where chronic illness symptoms are already experienced as high and psychological well-being is low, the platform is described as floundering. Positive psychological interventions with persons who are currently languishing or floundering would aim to extend the person's current coping competencies in order to make psychological well-being goals more attainable. A measure of stabilisation and resilience might then be achieved if that person can hold onto their home, relationships and roles, that is, the 'good things in life'.

A person with high psychological well-being who is also encountering high levels of chronic illness symptoms could be seen to be adapting. That person might still be vulnerable to a collapse of adaptation success in the event of any surge in environmental demands (e.g. stress as a result of relocation away from home, or non-desired change in relationships or roles). Where chronic illness symptoms are experienced as low, whilst psychological well-being is high, the person is on a platform we may refer to as *flourishing*. Positive psychological interventions with persons who are currently *adapting* or *flourishing* would strengthen and extend the person's existing coping competencies, further fostering resilience in advance of any further adverse events.

HOW WELL-BEING CAN BE PRESERVED FOR PEOPLE LIVING WITH CHRONIC ILLNESS IN LATER LIFE

Illnesses and/or changed abilities will be experienced by all of us at some point in our lives. The question is not how we avoid these but rather how well we live with such challenges and possibly curtailed resources.

Understanding the processes that underlie the capacity to cope and adapt well naturally provides valuable insights for planning interventions, where these are needed, to protect well-being. There is an increasing interest in the development of PP interventions that are based on this premise to improve quality of life in ageing. For example, Ramirez *et al.* (2014) developed an intervention that selected positive life review, forgiveness and gratitude as three PP factors linked with well-being in later life. Participants were aged 60–93 years and those with health problems were not excluded from the study. The intervention comprised 90-minute group sessions held weekly for nine weeks and this was shown to be sufficient in decreasing anxiety and depression as well as improving life satisfaction and happiness (see Ramirez *et al.*, 2014).

Work to understand the processes underlying how people cope well in illness-related adversity in later life has yielded other key constructs, captured here as resilience, optimism and positive expectancy and self-efficacy.

RESILIENCE

Resilience might be defined as 'the capacity for successful adaptation, positive functioning, or competence despite high risk, chronic stress, or prolonged or severe trauma' (Henry, 1999, p.521). Resilience is seen as a naturally occurring phenomenon in the individual that will naturally prevail unless specific conditions occur. Treating people as a member of a group that is less valued in society is the force most likely to overwhelm individual resilience. By implication, this opens up the possibility that every individual, irrespective of age, can protect their resilience through the life-span by resisting the internalisation of negative stereotypes and positively valuing the experience of later life.

There are several conditions necessary for fostering resilience (Cheston and Bender, 1999; Gilligan, 2000). These include:

- a sense of a secure base (attachment/networks with responsive people and continuity in life patterns)

- self-esteem (secure harmonious relationships and attention to wider life goals related to one's own interests)

- a sense of agency (having internal regulation over one's own life conditions and decisions).

Accordingly, promoting or protecting these conditions in the experience of the person in later life living with chronic illness is likely to foster and boost natural resilience (also see Chapter 6, this volume).

The application of PP to health has aided identification of key concepts to help explain how some people retain resilience to achieve positive adjustment, while others develop symptoms of stress in the context of life-defining long-term health conditions. Constructing a sense of *meaningfulness* about the circumstances appears to be a core process, helping to replace the sense of chaos with *understanding* and to replace the sense of intolerability with *coping*. Positive beliefs tie in with this; being able to derive different meanings in reaction to the threat of illness has been consistently linked with adjustment to and recovery from a range of chronic conditions (see Taylor and Sherman, 2004 for a review). Similarly, finding *benefit* in adversity and experiencing *growth* in the aftermath of trauma are surprisingly common among people experiencing life-defining illnesses. Benefit finding, in particular, has been linked with lowered psychological distress and more adaptive health behaviours across chronic and terminal illnesses, and it has also been shown to be amenable to psychological intervention (e.g. see Stanton *et al.*, 2002).

OPTIMISM AND POSITIVE EXPECTANCY

Dispositional optimism – involving the global belief that more desirable than undesirable things will occur in the future – is associated with better coping with a variety of health challenges, including better recovery from cardiovascular surgery (Scheier *et al.*, 1989) and improved survival rates with cancer (Allison, Fung and Gilain, 2003). Higher levels of optimism tend also to be associated with other positive cognitive and behavioural factors, including: a capacity to use *flexible* adaptive strategies, a tendency to be *approach-oriented* and a perceived personal capacity to *control stressors*. As we saw earlier (Urry and Gross, 2010), increases in emotion regulation can enhance such capacities in later life.

Positive expectancy also relates to the power of societal beliefs about individuals or groups in society (e.g. people in later life) to make it more likely that those individuals will have a positive experience of their lives and a positive image in their own and others' eyes. Evidence now accumulating within PP opens up an array of positive expectancies about later life (e.g. continuing development, well-being, wisdom and emancipation). Positive expectancies about people promote valued social roles, which, as we have seen, are protective of self-esteem and a buffer against adverse events. Positive expectancy also provides a counter to those negative societal expectancies about later life such as 'past it', 'a burden', 'diminishing powers' and suchlike, which can result in individuals acting down to negative beliefs, weak social roles and demoralisation about later life (Kitwood, 1997).

A major impact of chronic illness can be framed as 'secondary and tertiary impairment' (in the terms of SRV). Where a person is seen as different from the norm, perhaps because of a disability or by being seen as closer to death, there is the risk of that person being seen as less of a person and therefore denied socially valued roles. This leads to the erosion of relationships and roles and ultimately to the person internalising a view of themselves as unworthy and a burden. Impairments therefore not only arise from the impact of chronic health conditions but also from the impact of internalised negative images and assumptions. Building useful and positive beliefs and expectations about ageing (i.e. based on evidence about positive developments and experience) is an intervention likely to have a positive impact on health and well-being. Damaging and distorted beliefs about chronic illness in later life can pervade – for example: 'I wouldn't want to live if I had X so I don't think people with X want to live.' The counter might be: 'Later life provides opportunities for dealing with new challenges in new ways. People in later life who are dealing with chronic illness and other adversities are valued by succeeding generations. They are admired for how they inspire others, set an example, feel certain about what is worthwhile and live in a way that is free from earlier life pre-occupations and limitations.'

SELF-EFFICACY

Self-efficacy concerns the belief that one has the capability to perform actions that will positively influence events and outcomes that are personally important. Levels of self-efficacy are associated with positive coping with adverse events (Bandura, 2001) and better health in later life (Grembowski *et al.*, 1993). The processes by which self-efficacy supports health and well-being include the following: *goal setting* is used as a coping approach; *self-agency thoughts* are deployed; and limitations tend to be seen as *opportunities* (Klausner, Snyder and Cheavens, 2000). Like resilience, self-efficacy may accrue naturally over the course of the life-span and there is evidence that it continues into later life (Penninx *et al.*, 1998). Self-efficacy interventions aim to strengthen the perception that it is possible to act positively (e.g. engage in exercise) on outcomes that are salient and desirable (reducing body weight). Simultaneously, they aim to minimise circumstances in which we label a person as having a 'poor quality of life' – a construct that can be harmful if applied from the viewpoint of earlier adult life. Knowing as we do now that later life brings transformative changes in values, it follows that a person's sense of self-efficacy is underpinned in later life by developing a new vista of competencies and self-image. PP points to the pivotal roles of secure relationships, transcendent life goals and internal regulation as being important in promoting strong self-efficacy beliefs in later life. By the same token, environments and communities that have the capacity to enhance self-efficacy in later life will potentially be inspirational for people across the life-span.

INTEGRATION AND SUMMARY

PP offers a framework for understanding flourishing and how it might occur even in the context of later life and the experience of health-related adversity. A PP perspective encourages us to focus explicitly on what is still going right as we encounter illnesses and as we age. Positive states and experiences have real benefits in relation to health and well-being and potentially represent the transformation of personal meanings. PP also carries the important principle that positive and negative states are not simply opposite ends of the same continuum. As such, so called 'second-wave' approaches to PP (see Lomas and Ivtzan, 2015) emphasise a dialectical understanding of well-being, one that involves an interplay between the positive and negative experiences in which negative processes (e.g. adversity) may lead to positive outcomes (e.g. meaning and growth). Such processes and outcomes also need to be seen in context. These approaches are highly relevant to understanding how well-being and flourishing might be attained in the face of age-associated physical and psychological challenges and, as we have seen, several particular positive factors (e.g. gerotranscendence, optimism, resilience, growth) have been linked both with well-being in ageing and positive adaptation to chronic health problems. As we go forward there is still much to learn about how different components of well-being (e.g. PERMA) are sustained in experiences of ageing and illness, and how they might interact.

Far from inevitably resulting in loss and misery, later life can often bring positive changes that contribute to increased well-being. These are underpinned by processes such as a transformation in values, an increased focus on what is personally meaningful and emancipation from previous psychological and social boundaries. The term 'cosmic transcendence' has been used to capture the experience of liberation and connection with life that widely occurs with ageing. It is described as a sense of being a key contributing part of the whole system of life. Later life has been reported to bring unprecedented development of the capacities for reflection, future focus, responsiveness in relationships and increasing self-esteem and fulfilment. As such, profiles of personal strengths can be enhanced as people develop across the life-span. Whilst there is still much to learn about the domains of positive functioning that might contribute most to well-being in ageing and in the experience of illness, individuals of all ages potentially have much to gain from sharing life experiences and interacting with people in later life.

We have seen how interventions based on PP have the potential to enhance well-being in later life and in the experience of long-term health problems. Accessing specific, positive autobiographical memories enhances well-being; accepting and forgiving the deficits of transgressors increases self-esteem and hope; perceiving events as gifts increases well-being and repairs mood in the aftermath of trauma (Ramirez *et al.*, 2014). In a more general sense, individual personal futures planning in the context of chronic life-defining disability has long been recognised as increasing well-being for both the focal person and those people who are gifted new and fulfilling life-support roles (O'Brien and Lovett, 1992). It can also be argued that well-being and coping with adversity are most effectively achieved when society enables the widest possible development in all individuals of the pro-social skills of '*looking after each other*' (Smail, 2001). This highlights the social context of well-being across the life-span and indicates again that community-level interventions are indicated in enhancing the congruence between the abilities and assets of the person and the demands and resources in the environment in order to enhance security, stability and quality of life (Ranzijn, 2002).

Later life fulfils a unique purpose in the cycle of life, bringing opportunities for the development of positive humanitarian competencies and freedom from the material and production concerns that dominate earlier adult life. This is not to deny that later life is accompanied by increasingly likely encounters with chronic illness and life-defining disabilities. Chronic health challenges, however, can open up an array of opportunities never before experienced, including for reciprocal relationships, certainty about what is meaningful, satisfaction with what is present in life, and a sense of connection and place. The capacity of individuals in later life to potentially flourish and grow strong while living with adversity may have an important bearing on the imminent and pressing question of how humans across the life-span will succeed in adapting happily to global environmental challenges. In the current context of ecological imperatives, society is looking for ways to develop human resilience and happiness across the full extent of the extending adult life-span. Identifying and maximising the processes that enable flourishing in later life may hold significance for our development of social progress world-wide.

REFERENCES

Allison, P.J, Fung, K. and Gilain, L. (2003) 'Dispositional optimism predicts survival status 1 year after diagnosis in head and neck cancer patients.' *Journal of Clinical Oncology 21*(3), 543–548.

Aspinwall, L.G. and Tedeschi, R.G. (2010) 'The value of positive psychology for health psychology: Progress and pitfalls in examining the relation of positive phenomena to health.' *Annals of Behavioral Medicine 39*, 4–15.

Bandura, A. (2001) 'The changing face of psychology at the dawning of a globalisation era.' *Canadian Psychology 42*(1), 12–24.

Bergland, Å., and Kirkevold, M. (2006) 'Thriving in nursing homes in Norway: contributing aspects described by residents.' *International Journal of Nursing Studies 43*(6), 681–691.

Cheston, R. and Bender, M. (1999) *Understanding Dementia: The Man with the Worried Eyes.* London: Jessica Kingsley Publishers.

Cosco, T.D., Prina, A.M., Perales, J., Stephan, B. and Brayne, C. (2014) 'Operational definitions of successful aging: A systematic review.' *International Psychogeriatrics 26*(3), 373–381.

Diener, E. and Suh, E.M. (1998) 'Subjective Well-being and Age: An International Analysis.' In K.W. Schaie and M.P. Lawton (eds) *Annual Review of Gerontology and Geriatrics (Vol. 17).* New York: Springer.

Flynn, R.J. and Lemay, R.A. (1999) *A Quarter Century of Normalisation and Social Role Valorization: Evolution and Impact.* Ottawa: University of Ottawa Press.

Frederickson, B.L. (2004) 'The broaden-and-build theory of positive emotions.' *Philosophical Transactions of the Royal Society B: Biological Sciences 359*, 1367–1377.

Fredrickson, B.L. and Losada, M.F. (2005) 'Positive affect and the complex dynamics of human flourishing.' *American Psychologist 60*(7), 678.

Gilligan, R. (2000) 'Adversity, resilience and young people: The protective value of positive school and spare time experiences.' *Children and Society 14*, 37–47.

Grembowski, D., Patrick, D., Diehr, P., Durham, M. *et al.* (1993) 'Self-efficacy and health behavior among older adults.' *Journal of Health and Social Behavior 34*(2), 89–104.

Haight B.K., Barba B.E., Tesh A.S. and Courts N.F. (2002) 'Thriving: a life span theory.' *Journal of Gerontological Nursing 28*(3), 14–22.

Henry, D.L. (1999) 'Resilience in maltreated children: Implications for special needs adoption.' *Child Welfare 78*(5), 519–540.

Helliwell, R., Layard, J. and Sachs, J. (2015) *World Happiness Report 2015.* UN: Sustainable Development Solutions Network. Available at http://worldhappiness.report/wp-content/uploads/sites/2/2015/04/WHR15.pdf, accessed on 9 May 2016.

Kern, M.L., Waters, L.E., Adler, A. and White, M.A. (2015) 'A multidimensional approach to measuring well-being in students: Application of the PERMA framework.' *The Journal of Positive Psychology 10*(3), 262–271.

Keyes, C.L. (2007) 'Promoting and protecting mental health as flourishing: a complementary strategy for improving national mental health.' *American Psychologist 62*(2), 95–108.

Keyes, C.L.M. and Lopez, S.J. (2005) 'Toward a Science of Mental Health.' In C.R. Snyder and S.J. Lopez (eds) *Handbook of Positive Psychology.* Oxford: Oxford University Press.

Kok, A.A., Aartsen, M.J., Deeg, D.J. and Huisman, M. (2015) 'Capturing the diversity of successful aging: An operational definition based on 16-year trajectories of functioning.' *The Gerontologist.* DOI: 10.1093/geront/gnv127

Kitwood, T. (1997) *Dementia Reconsidered.* Milton Keynes: Open University Press.

Klausner, E., Snyder, C.R. and Cheavens, J. (2000) 'A Hope Based Group Treatment for Depressed Older Outpatients.' In G.M. Williamson, P.A. Parmalee and D.R. Shaffer (eds) *Physical Illness and Depression in Older Adults.* New York: Plenum.

Lemay, R. (1999) 'Roles, Identities and Expectancies: Positive Contributions of Role Theory to Normalization and Social Role Valorization.' In R.J. Flynn and R.A. Lemay (eds) *A Quarter Century of Normalization and Social Role Valorization: Evolution and Impact.* Ottawa, ON: University of Ottawa Press.

Linley, P.A. and Joseph, S. (2004) *Positive Psychology in Practice.* Hoboken, NJ: Wiley.

Lockenhoff, C.E. and Carstensen, L.L. (2004) 'Balance between regulating emotions and making tough choices.' *Journal of Personality 72*(6), 1395–1424.

Lomas, T. (2016) 'The Dialectics of Emotion.' In I. Ivtzan , T. Lomas, K. Hefferon and P. Worth (eds) *Second Wave Positive Psychology – Embracing the Dark Side of Life.* Abingdon: Routledge.

Lomas, T. and Ivtzan, I. (2015) 'Second wave positive psychology: Exploring the positive–negative dialectics of wellbeing.' *Journal of Happiness Studies.* Available at http://hdl.handle.net/10552/4383, accessed on 23 October 2015.

Malone, J.C., Cohen, S., Liu, S.R., Vaillant, G.E. and Waldinger, R.J. (2013) 'Adaptive midlife defense mechanisms and late-life health.' *Personality and Individual Differences 55*(2), 85–89.

O'Brien, J. and Lovett, H. (1992) *Finding a Way Toward Everyday Lives: The Contribution of Person Centered Planning.* Harrisburg, PA: Pennsylvania Office of Mental Retardation.

Penninx, B.W., Guralnik, J.M., Simonsick, E.M., Kasper, J.D., Ferrucci, L. and Fried, L.P. (1998) 'Emotional vitality among disabled older women: The Women's Health and Aging Study.' *Journal of the American Geriatrics Society 46*, 807–815.

Peterson, C. and Park, N. (2009) 'Classifying and Measuring Strengths of Character.' In S.J. Lopez and C.R. Snyder (eds) *The Oxford Handbook of Positive Psychology.* New York: Oxford University Press.

Peterson, C. and Seligman, M.E.P. (2004) *Character Strengths and Virtues: A Handbook of Classification.* Washington, DC: Oxford University Press.

Ramirez, E., Ortega, A.R., Chamorro, A. and Colmenero J.M. (2014) 'A program of positive intervention in the elderly: Memories, gratitude and forgiveness.' *Aging and Mental Health 18*(4), 463–470.

Ranzijn, R. (2002) 'The potential of older adults to enhance community quality of life: Links between positive psychology and productive aging.' *Ageing International* 27(2), 30–55.

Rosling, H. (2015) *Don't panic – the facts about population*. A one-hour long documentary broadcast on BBC on 7 November 2013. Available at www.gapminder.org/videos/dont-panic-the-facts-about-population, accessed on 14 April 2016.

Rusk, R.D. and Waters, L. (2014) 'A psycho-social system approach to well-being: Empirically deriving the Five Domains of Positive Functioning.' *The Journal of Positive Psychology 9*, 1–12.

Scheier, M.F., Matthews, K.A., Owens, J.F., Magovern G.J. *et al.* (1989) 'Dispositional optimism and recovery from coronary artery bypass surgery: The beneficial effects on physical and psychological well-being.' *Journal of Personal Social Psychology 57*, 1024–1040.

Schueller, S.M., Jayawickreme, E., Blackie, L.E., Forgeard, M.J. and Roepke, A.M. (2015) 'Finding character strengths through loss: An extension of Peterson and Seligman (2003).' *The Journal of Positive Psychology 10*(1), 53–63.

Seligman, M.E. (1999) 'The president's address.' *American Psychologist 54*(8), 559–562.

Seligman, M.E.P. (2005) 'Positive Psychology, Positive Prevention and Positive Therapy.' In C.R. Snyder and S.J. Lopez (eds) *Handbook of Positive Psychology*. New York: Oxford University Press.

Seligman, M.E.P. (2011) *Flourish: A Visionary New Understanding of Happiness and Well-being*. New York: NY: Simon and Schuster.

Smail, D. (2001) *Why Therapy Doesn't Work and What We Should Do about It*. London: Robinson.

Smith, W.J. (2003) *Forced Exit: The Slippery Slope from Assisted Suicide to Legalized Murder*. Dallas, TX: Spence Publishing Company.

Stanton, A.L., Danoff-Burg, S., Sworowski, L.A., Collins, C.A. *et al.* (2002) 'Randomized, controlled trial of written emotional expression and benefit finding in breast cancer patients.' *Journal of Clinical Oncology 20*(20), 4160–4168.

Stirling, E. (2010) *Valuing Older People: Positive Psychological Practice*. Chichester: John Wiley and Sons Ltd.

Sudnow, D. (1967) *Passing On: The Social Organisation of Dying*. New Jersey, NJ: Prentice-Hall.

Taylor, S.E. and Sherman, D.K. (2004) 'Positive Psychology and Health Psychology: A Fruitful Liaison.' In P.A. Linley and S. Joseph (eds) *Positive Psychology in Practice*. Hoboken, NJ: Wiley.

Tornstam, L. (2011) 'Maturing into gerotranscendence.' *The Journal of Transpersonal Psychology 43*(2), 166–179.

Urry, H.L. and Gross, J.J. (2010) 'Emotion regulation in older age.' *Current Directions in Psychological Science 19*(6), 352–357.

Vaillant, G.E. (2004) 'Positive Ageing.' In P.A. Linley and S. Joseph (eds) *Positive Psychology in Practice*. Hoboken, NJ: Wiley.

Williamson, G. (2005) 'Aging Well: Outlook for the 21st Century.' In C.R. Snyder and S.J. Lopez (eds) *Handbook of Positive Psychology*. Oxford: Oxford University Press.

Wolfensberger, W. (1998) *A Brief Introduction to Social Role Valorization as a Higher Order Concept for Addressing the Plight of Societally Devalued People, and for Structuring Human Services*. New York, NY: Training Institute for Human Service Planning, Leadership and Change Agentry, Syracuse University.

Wolfensberger, W. (2000) 'A brief overview of social role valorization.' *Mental Retardation 38*, 105–123.

Wong, P.T.P. (2011) 'Positive psychology 2.0: Towards a balanced interactive model of the good life.' *Canadian Psychology 52*(2), 69–81.

Worth, P. (2016) 'Positive Development – Our Journey.' In I. Ivtzan, T. Lomas, K. Hefferon and P. Worth (eds) *Second Wave Positive Psychology – Embracing the Dark Side of Life*. Abingdon: Routledge.

Wrzesniewski, A. (2005) 'Jobs, Careers and Callings.' In C.R. Snyder and S.J. Lopez (eds) *Handbook of Positive Psychology*. New York, NY: Oxford University Press.

Chapter 2

A POSITIVE PSYCHOLOGY APPROACH TO DEMENTIA

Chris Clarke, Emma Wolverson and Esme Moniz-Cook

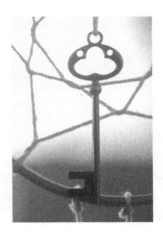

Taking a positive perspective on living with dementia may appear profoundly counter-intuitive. Media accounts, academic texts and scientific research usually speak of how intensely challenging dementia can be, how care services are stretched almost to breaking point and how dementia represents an enormous social and economic burden to society. Yet, at the same time, in our work with people who live with dementia we regularly encounter laughter, enjoyment and awe – as we bear witness to the personal strengths, positive meanings and deep connections that people preserve as they strive to live as well as is possible. These experiences may not be shared by all. However, without deliberate and thoughtful inquiry into their extent and nature, the voices of those who do have such experiences will not be heard and the knowledge base arising from what they have to teach us will be much the poorer.

Accordingly, this chapter explores the potential for applying positive psychology approaches (described in Chapter 1) to widening our understanding of the experience of living with dementia, in its varying forms. Central to this chapter are the factors that might comprise and sustain well-being and optimal functioning in dementia, from the point of view of those living with it.

A positive psychological approach to dementia emphasises the continuing presence of positive abilities, assets and resources as people strive to maintain their selfhood. However, in order to develop the case for looking beyond loss and pathology towards a positive psychology conceptualisation of living with dementia, a critical appraisal of the dominant disease-based narrative around the condition is first outlined. This prevailing narrative has historically centred on pathology, decline and loss or stigmatising social processes. Here, it is described first in order to demonstrate its stark contrast with the aspirations of a positive psychology of dementia, since these differences must be clearly understood from the outset.

DEMENTIA – THE NARRATIVE OF DISEASE

How dementia is lived with remains subject to powerful clinical, social and political discourses within which biomedical accounts have formed a dominant narrative. In this narrative, the language we use is typically reductionist, clinical and technical. The word 'dementia' is primarily constructed as a neurodegenerative syndrome with discernible biological causes (e.g. Alzheimer's disease) that manifest in progressive changes in a person's cognitive and functional capabilities. A purely biomedical approach to dementia research and practice, described as the 'standard paradigm' by Kitwood (1997), assumes a straightforward relationship between the type and extent of cerebral damage and the signs and symptoms of the condition (e.g. memory loss, impaired judgement, functional decline and so on). Within this approach, dementia is understood primarily as a biological disorder with defined symptoms and stages that leads inexorably to loss of function and end-of-life.

This account of dementia has been dominant at both clinical and popular levels of discourse, possibly because it resonates with increasing technological dependence in most Western societies (Stirling, 2010), in which it is believed that illness, framed in terms of disease, can ultimately be conquered via technological advances. Thus, hope in dementia rests solely on finding a medical cure. It is a model that has underpinned developments in health policies and the growth of dementia advocacy movements, including those promoted by the world-wide Alzheimer societies. It sustains pharmaceutical companies engaged in the search for a cure, as it directs both political attention and much-needed financial resources towards this endeavour. Undoubtedly, these efforts represent positive intentions – the prevention and alleviation of the suffering that can arise from dementia is arguably one of the greatest technical, clinical and societal challenges of the 21st century, and improving awareness, engagement, treatment and care in dementia have become global priorities (World Health Organization, 2015). However, an exclusively biomedical and disease-based account of dementia can (and should) be challenged on philosophical, humanistic and empirical grounds.

First, this model of dementia can be viewed as a technologically based Western social construction of ageing and health that carries implicit assumptions about what makes for a happy and successful life. Such social constructions are abstract social concepts that develop and are sustained through language and shared beliefs (e.g. that it is not possible to sustain well-being if one is living with dementia), which are themselves socio-politically situated. They do not therefore represent 'psychological facts about people' (Maddux, 2009, p.63), but might be mistaken for them.

Second, biomedical discourses also maintain a restricted social construction of the *experience* of dementia that itself becomes a source of personal suffering for those living with the condition. Dementia is reported to be the most feared illness amongst the general public (see Brunet *et al.*, 2012). At its worst, dementia is constructed as a 'living death' (see Behuniak, 2011). Military metaphors are used persuasively to depict dementia as an enemy to do battle with and defeat. However, such narratives become connected with the negative stereotyping of people with dementia, who are often depicted as helpless 'victims' or 'sufferers' and who have little hope of leading a meaningful life until the 'miracle cure' has been discovered. This in turn weakens the validity of approaches based upon good care and rehabilitation, and limits the agency that people with dementia are seen to be able to exercise (see George and Whitehouse, 2014). This stereotyping can also influence the beliefs of a person with dementia, in that an assumed loss of all capabilities, including the self and identity, can become internalised as a self-stereotype (Scholl and Sabat, 2008) as one progresses to become regarded as a form of 'zombie' (Behuniak, 2011). Thus, internalised negative emotions such as fear and disgust undermine positive emotions and hopefulness for people with dementia as well their loved ones. Mitchell, Dupuis and Kontos (2013) describe how fear-based metaphors and images, underpinned by biomedical discourses around dementia, contribute to a powerful *othering* process in which the embodied selfhood of a person is effectively disregarded. They highlight how depersonalising care practices and even entire organisational cultures are potentially reciprocally linked with this process, thus perpetuating an assumed loss of identity as well as increased distress for people living with dementia.

Third, several authorities have drawn attention to the multiplicity of causes and presentations in dementia and the lack of a linear relationship between brain pathology and levels of ability. Whitehouse (2008) challenges the accepted validity of Alzheimer's-type dementia as a classifiable disease by highlighting the lack of a consistent correlation between the presence and level of beta-amyloid protein plaques apparent at post-mortem and the level of cognitive impairment people have experienced. Karran, Mercken and De Strooper (2011) argue that, so far, attempts to treat Alzheimer's disease by pharmacologically reducing beta-amyloid have been largely unsuccessful and in some cases even harmful, prompting searching questions about its assumed causative role. Portacolone *et al.* (2014) note that both neural plaques and cerebro-vascular changes occur commonly in *normal* human ageing, suggesting that dementia lies on a continuum with cognitive ageing rather than being a classifiable disease-based phenomenon.

These views form part of a counter-narrative about the nature and experience of dementia that has been steadily emerging. In this narrative, dementia is framed as a bio-psycho-social condition (see Spector and Orrell, 2010) where biophysical, psychological and socio-cultural factors interact to determine when and how vulnerable individuals encounter progressive cognitive impairments as they age. In this frame, people are viewed as remaining active within their experiences of dementia (Clare, 2002), possessing universal human desires to experience well-being, autonomy and positive relationships. Dementia therefore overlaps with dimensions of normal human ageing, and a bio-psycho-social approach can also incorporate some of the understandings of successful ageing that were outlined in Chapter 1. An important focus of the physical health component of a bio-psycho-social approach is that of the timely management of co-morbid health conditions, such as infection, heart disease, diabetes, or symptoms due to drug interactions, as they occur in a person with dementia. Such conditions have previously been ignored when changes in the person's behaviour were mis-attributed to progression of the dementia; this therefore undermined the well-being of the person.

BEYOND THE DISEASE NARRATIVE – TOWARDS A POSITIVE PSYCHOLOGY APPROACH

Two major themes from the dementia literature signify the potential application of positive psychology to living with dementia. The first concerns individual identity and its preservation in the face of cognitive change. Within this, attention to positive subjective experiences, personal strengths and the quality of relationships is paramount. The second concerns the use and influence of language in relation to how dementia is perceived and experienced within society.

THE PERSON-CENTRED PERSPECTIVE

Kitwood and Bredin (1992) first introduced a psycho-social theory of dementia care in which the unfolding experience of dementia involves an interplay between neuropathology, a person's biography and personality, and the social psychology around them. Central to this approach is the concept of personhood; a moral status that is afforded within social relationships and in which someone is seen as unique, possessing agency and being intrinsically worthy of respect (Kitwood, 1997). This theory places the preservation of personhood, which does not and should not rest upon a person's cognitive status (see Post, 2013), as a central concern in maintaining positive well-being. The expression of personhood in dementia is perhaps primarily an embodied, physical experience and the preservation of personhood in dementia care is therefore critically linked with the capacity of the social environment to be positively responsive to an embodied sense of self and personal identity (see Kontos and Martin, 2013). Personhood therefore has dynamic qualities with the 'potential to evolve' (Dewing, 2008, p.5) insofar as social environments and, arguably, public discourses can facilitate this.

Pivotally, in describing a theory of personhood in dementia, Kitwood and Bredin (1992) also introduced the notion that relative well-being in dementia manifests behaviourally and has 12 observable indicators. Several of these relate directly to positive psychology concepts such as the ability to experience and display positive emotion, humour, creativity and compassion for others. Moreover, they proposed that well-being in dementia is underpinned by the achievement and preservation of four global, subjective states that represent core psychological needs. These are described in terms of a sense of personal worth, a sense of personal agency, a feeling of being of use to and accepted by others, and having hope that personal needs for psychological security will continue to be met. Kitwood and Bredin's theoretical position focused on how the social environment around the person with dementia should be attentive to and foster these global subjective psychological states and associated needs, in order to support and maintain the person's emotional well-being and quality of life.

CONNECTIONS WITH POSITIVE PSYCHOLOGY

Principles and concepts from positive psychology complement a person-centred approach to dementia in several key ways. In rejecting a pure 'illness ideology' (Maddux, 2009), the starting point in positive psychology is to inquire about what is working, what remains and what is right in our lives that allows us to experience positive well-being. Applied to dementia, this perspective underlines the importance of highlighting and preserving wellness, rather than treating illness. This notion is part of the philosophy of person-centred care and underpins tools such as Dementia Care Mapping (see Brooker and Surr, 2005), but positive psychology brings an additional layer of valuable concepts and perspectives on what well-being is and how it might be attained within the context of the challenges and constraints that arise from the condition. Thus, positive psychology models of well-being and flourishing have the potential to inform person-centred approaches to dementia and this can be conceptually illustrated in four ways:

- *Subjective versus psychological well-being:* A distinction can be drawn between two forms of well-being. Subjective, hedonic well-being relates to life satisfaction and the experience of positive and negative emotions in the moment. In contrast, psychological or eudemonic well-being refers to a process of pursuing meaningful goals and having a sense of purpose in spite of life's challenges. Both forms of well-being are of relevance to living well with dementia and implicitly underpin the person-centred approach, but an explicit focus on how these might be experienced by people living with dementia has yet to take place. In the context of dementia there remains much to learn about how these two aspects of well-being interact, how they manifest behaviourally and how each can be best supported by social environments (see Chapter 3).

- *Models of well-being-process and outcome:* Dodge and colleagues (2012) define well-being in terms a dynamic interplay between the challenges a person is facing versus the physical, psychological and social resources at their disposal. This approach highlights how a certain level of challenge is necessary to achieve well-being, but it must also be balanced against the person's resources, which in turn must be accessible and flexible enough to meet challenges. In dementia, achieving such a balance is crucial. For example, some level of positive challenge – perhaps in the form of cognitive stimulation – is beneficial (Spector *et al.*, 2003), yet it is also vital that a person's resources are protected and enabled, so that challenges can be met and well-being achieved (see Chapter 6). As an outcome, well-being is likely to be multi-dimensional and this is also of relevance to conceptualising well-being in dementia, where the meeting of intersecting psychological needs is vital. Seligman's (2011) PERMA approach to well-being, for example, highlights how positive emotions, engagement, relationships, meaning and accomplishment might combine to determine flourishing. Helping people to realise these outcomes simultaneously would be central to a positive person-centred approach to dementia.

- *Domains of positive functioning:* Rusk and Waters' (2014) empirical model of the processes underpinning positive functioning draws further attention to the notion of multiple pathways to achieving well-being. It highlights different aspects or forms of positive functioning that potentially interact in idiosyncratic ways, depending on a person's context and resources. Applied to dementia, this model suggests that preserving resources or providing support in one domain of functioning, such as positive emotions and relationships, may well have a positive impact on others, such as 'comprehension and coping' (see Chapter 12 for a further exploration of the application of this model to well-being in dementia).

- *Affect Balance:* Rather than reflecting the simple presence or absence of positive and negative emotions, Fredrickson and Losada (2005) demonstrate how well-being relates to the relative balance or ratio between the two. A person may well experience negative states and emotions but if this is sufficiently outweighed by positive states and experiences on a daily basis then they are more likely to be able to move toward a state of flourishing. Kolanowski and colleagues (2014) tested the applicability of this conceptualisation of well-being to dementia, amongst 128 care home residents living with the condition. Those participants who had high levels of overall well-being (approximately 10% of the sample) had a positive/negative affect ratio of around 2.21 (i.e. just over 2 instances of positive emotion for every instance of negative emotion, over a 20-minute period). This ratio was significantly different to that of people who had low or moderate levels of well-being and the ratio predicted levels of engagement in activity. Such findings highlight how improving the balance of negative and positive emotions, in connection with activity engagement, might improve well-being in dementia.

Recognising and valuing individual differences in the way people experience and respond to cognitive and functional change would be intrinsic to a positive psychology-informed approach, allowing for the potential influence of personal strengths, such as perseverance, and adaptive personality traits, such as openness, on the experience of well-being. Individual differences will also, inevitably, be reflective of the extent to which social environments enable people to maintain choice, agency and connection in their lives. These processes relate closely to the notion of self-determination (Wehmeyer, Little and Sergeant, 2009), a key positive psychology approach to understanding human agency, motivation and well-being that has, thus far, been an under-developed element of person-centred approaches to dementia. Self-determination theory (Deci and Ryan, 2002) contends that people actively seek to meet and achieve integration between three fundamental psychological needs – *competence* (the need to have mastery and be effective in one's environment) and *autonomy* (being able to act in accordance with one's personal goals and values) on the one hand, and *relatedness* (the need for connectedness and belonging) on the other. For any person, well-being is likely to be optimised when these needs are achieved in balance and where social contexts enable this. There is a high degree of overlap between this perspective and person-centred models of well-being in dementia (cf. Kitwood, 1997), highlighting not only the universality of the link between psychological needs and positive well-being but also how people with dementia are likely to retain an active motivation to fulfil such needs. Conceptualisations of agency from a positive psychology perspective can therefore inform and refine person-centred approaches in dementia.

THE POWER OF LANGUAGE

Positive psychology is rooted in the premise that well-being is subject to the quality of positive relationships and social contexts, including socio-cultural narratives. This is also central to person-centred and relational accounts of dementia care (see Chapter 10). Language and discourse shape how we frame dementia and how people's experiences of dementia are understood and interacted with. Attending to the potential to change such language is central to fostering a narrative of hope – that people living with dementia are capable of having meaningful positive experiences and retaining personal strengths.

The social narratives available to people living *without* dementia, perhaps particularly in developed nations, by default, involve a language of aspiration, competence, mastery and fulfilment. These concepts and values are also interwoven with positive psychology. However, historical stereotypes and stigma mean that these narratives have not been accessible for people living with dementia, even if their personal experiences and goals might continue to comprise such themes. As Harris and Keady (2008) note, discourses surrounding dementia have seldom involved the deliberate use of positive terms such as resilience, wisdom and successful ageing. Until recently, using such terms in relation to living with dementia would have appeared counter-intuitive. Yet, the potential benefits of pairing such language with the experience of dementia present new and hugely encouraging avenues for research and practice in relation to living well.

Correspondingly, there are now increasing international efforts to *upgrade* public discourses in favour of de-stigmatising dementia, reducing fear of the condition and ending discrimination at community and societal levels. These initiatives focus both on socially re-contextualising the meaning of dementia and on making simultaneous positive attempts to improve knowledge and perceptions surrounding the condition. This movement is connected with broader and ongoing efforts to create 'dementia-friendly' communities, which are now an international social phenomenon adopted by the public-health policy makers of several nations. [1]

'LIVING WELL' WITH DEMENTIA

Alongside dementia *friendliness*, further evidence of a shift in discourses lies in the adoption of the concept of 'living well' rather than simply 'living with' dementia (Rahman, 2014). In the UK, living well with dementia was first enshrined explicitly in health policy with the publication of the National Dementia Strategy for England (Department of Health, 2009), which set out how the strategic development of health and social care services should occur so as to improve the well-being of people living with dementia, as well as their families and caregivers. Subsequent health policy initiatives in the UK and beyond have continued to emphasise living well with dementia as a key objective, both in relation to national and local services and also research efforts (Department of Health, 2012).[2]

What does living well with dementia mean? Since a considerable body of research indicates that dementia confers a greater risk of depression, anxiety, long-term physical ill-health and social inequality

---

1 See www.alz.co.uk/dementia-friendly-communities
2 See www.alzheimer-europe.org/Policy-in-Practice2/National-Dementia-Plans

(see Alzheimer's disease International, 2012; Poblador-Plou *et al.*, 2014; Wragg and Jeste, 1989), it might be easy to dismiss living well as political rhetoric, borne out of a collective form of wishful thinking. Pertinently, a large opinion poll conducted in the UK in 2014 revealed that 43 per cent of adults surveyed believed that it is not possible to live a 'good life' with dementia and, in 2013, 54 per cent believed that quality of life for people with dementia is 'bad' or 'very bad' (Alzheimer's Society, 2014).

Previous academic research has also cast doubt on the notion that people living with dementia can have genuine positive experiences, with some suggesting that if positive experiences do occur they only represent a person's attempts to present a positive narrative to others in order to cope with loss and maintain a sense of personal and social value (see Steeman *et al.*, 2007). Thus, what might be genuine personal strengths and positive experiences for a person can become framed within existing discourses of loss, deficit and compensation, with the consequential narrative that it is not really possible to live positively with the condition being maintained.

However, living well is only beginning to be explored scientifically from the perspective of people who have dementia (see, for example, Clare *et al.*, 2014). Potentially, it is an organising concept for the notion that people can actively engage with and adjust to dementia, seek positive experiences and enjoy quality of life *in spite of* changes in physical, cognitive and daily living abilities (or be supported to do so), and can thus live with dementia in the background rather than the foreground of their lives. More controversially, perhaps, living well with dementia might also relate to the possibility of having positive experiences or displaying personal strengths *because of* the condition (see Chapter 7).

Do people living with dementia consider themselves to be able to live well? In 2013, the UK Alzheimer's Society surveyed 510 people living with dementia, 92 per cent of whom were continuing to live in the community (Kane and Cook, 2013). Whilst 63 per cent said that they felt anxious or depressed, 61 per cent reported that they were living well with dementia. This may appear contradictory, but positive psychology research shows how positive and negative experiences and emotions naturally co-occur and it is the balance between them that determines our overall levels of well-being across the life-span (see Diehl, Hay and Berg, 2011). This is pertinent if we link living with dementia to the experience of living with a chronic health condition of any kind, where traditional assumptions are that positive and negative experiences in illness are opposing and that positive adjustment to illness is only measurable in relation to the relative absence of negatives. Such a position can mean that people are not asked about their positive experiences in spite of being unwell and that having and reporting such experiences is seen as merely anomalous or else evidence of a failure to accept the condition (Aspinwall and Tedeschi, 2010).

Empirical work casts doubt on this way of understanding living with a long-term health condition. Paterson (2001), for example, on the basis of a review and analysis of 292 studies of living with a chronic illness, proposed that the personal salience of a long-term condition and its relative impact shifts dynamically over time according to the contexts and needs of the individual. This *shifting perspectives* account of living with a long-term health condition makes room for the distinct possibility that people's values, needs and relationships can continue to remain in the foreground of their lives and are not automatically subsumed under being unwell.

In examining the possibility that people living with dementia can live well, it is vital that we listen to how people describe their subjective experiences and perspectives. Historically, it was assumed that having dementia precludes the ability to form valid perceptions and judgements regarding the quality of one's life experiences. Clinicians and researchers tended to place weight on the views of caregivers or other proxies in determining the well-being of the person living with dementia. However, literature concerning the *lived experience* of dementia readily demonstrates that people have very meaningful things to say about various aspects of life with dementia, both positive and negative. This literature shows how the way dementia is perceived and responded to by those actually living with it involves an active and multi-faceted process of balancing loss and change with well-being and stability.

LIVED EXPERIENCES OF DEMENTIA: EMERGING EVIDENCE FOR POSITIVE PSYCHOLOGY CONCEPTUALISATIONS

In 2007, de Boer and colleagues conducted a systematic literature review of 50 studies of the subjective experience of living with dementia. Only studies that had described and explored aspects of dementia 'from the patient's [sic] perspective' were included. They identified two key themes in people's reported experiences of how they subjectively experienced the condition and its impact. These were *Impact* and *Coping*. The *Impact* of dementia referred to people's experiences of recognising, adjusting to and adapting to dementia and involves elements of loss and change in the context of relationships and care. *Coping* related to evidence that many people living with dementia actively use different coping strategies to adapt positively to the condition and its challenges. This is often based on a process of acceptance and coming to terms with the presence of dementia in one's life. Whilst the findings underline the challenges and negative impact of dementia, they also show that living with dementia involves active attempts to maintain self-determination, hope and well-being. Crucially, the authors highlight how their findings cast significant doubt on the assumption that dementia is inevitably a state of terrible suffering.

What people living with dementia themselves say about what they need to live well is a question of growing importance but, until recently, it has seldom been asked. The 'Good Life with Dementia' report, produced in conjunction with the UK Alzheimer's Society (see ESRO, 2014), was perhaps one of the first pieces of social research to shed light on this area. This ethnographic observational and interview-based research study involved people living with, or affected by, dementia and aimed to explore and determine what people define as important for their well-being, a process referred to as the 'makings of a good life'. Six broad themes emerged from this work, each pertaining to aspects of what might underpin living a good life in dementia, such as:

1. respecting identity and preserving selfhood
2. embracing experiences in the here and now
3. sustaining relationships
4. valuing contrasts (good days and bad days)
5. supporting agency
6. maintaining health.

It is striking, though perhaps not surprising, how these findings mirror both Kitwood and Bredin's (1992) original conceptualisation of well-being in dementia and also positive psychology constructs that are associated with psychological and subjective well-being, such as self-determination (see earlier), positive affect, the need for connectedness and positive relationships, resilience, and also the savouring of positive experiences in the present moment.

Our own work in this emerging area is concerned with how positive experiences and states might be experienced in dementia and how positive psychology approaches can be used to conceptualise these experiences. As a first step, we conducted a systematic review and synthesis of the dementia lived experience literature, including studies that reported on any kind of positive themes or experiences in the lives of older people with dementia (Wolverson, Clarke and Moniz-Cook, 2016). Twenty-six papers, published between 1992 and 2015, involving 422 people living with dementia across several different nations were included. Three key themes and nine sub-themes emerged from our synthesis of these studies' findings (see 'Themes' below).

The first major theme, *Engaging with Life in Ageing*, reflected people's positive approaches to the challenges of ageing, rather than dementia itself. Its three sub-themes collectively challenge the assumption that living with dementia is a wholly negative and devastating experience. Older people living with dementia may not organise and describe their experiences solely in relation to dementia but more with respect to their attempts to maintain their sense of agency as well as their experience of positive emotions and positive relationships as they age. These priorities, which are not far away from notions of successful ageing (see Chapter 1) can be in the foreground of people's experiences, with dementia somewhat in the background – an example of the shifting perspectives model of living with chronic health conditions described above (Paterson, 2001). Some may be able to place dementia in the background of their experiences because of preserved positive personality traits such as extraversion and openness to experience (Kolanowski, Litaker and Buettner, 2005). For others, maintaining engagement in meaningful and valued activities such as walking, music, reading, games and art (see Beard, 2004; Clare, Roth and Pratt, 2005) may be the key. Such activities may offer continued opportunities to experience in-the-moment well-being through *flow* (i.e. complete absorption in a meaningful task and its enjoyment) (Nakamura and Csikszentmihalyi, 2009; see also Chapter 8) despite dementia.

The second theme, *Engaging with Dementia*, and its three sub-themes, describe how people living with dementia draw on personal strengths to use active strategies aimed at maintaining well-being, continuity and positive relationships. Thus people with dementia might 'face and fight' the condition by taking an active decision to 'make the best' of life and not be defined or dominated by dementia and its challenges. For some, this comprised an explicit 'fight' against and rejection of dementia. For others, it appeared as a more subtle determination to continue to enjoy things and maintain their way of life in spite of dementia. A positive psychology perspective would help frame these experiences as examples of preserved personal strengths and virtues (Peterson and Seligman, 2004) in the context of living well with dementia. Examples of these strengths or virtues include: the capacity for *perspective* – using wisdom gained over one's life to 'look beyond' the dementia as part of accepting it (Clare, Goater and Woods, 2006); and *bravery* – using courage to face the challenges, threats and difficulties that dementia can bring (Harman and Clare, 2006).

The presence of *humour* and *hope* in people's experiences of dementia signifies how people might maintain well-being through the use of positive coping strategies that are also probably based on preserved personal strengths and capabilities. Thus, not only were people able to laugh and enjoy humour, they may deliberately use humour to diffuse the position and power of dementia in their everyday lives. Humour could also be important in maintaining close relationships in living with dementia (see Chapter 5). Similarly, hope is invoked with a sense of determination and agency and experienced as a crucial and generalised life force that supports well-being. It is also facilitated by positive relationships across the life-span (see Chapter 4).

The third theme, *Identity and Growth*, encompassed a higher level of personal, interpersonal and spiritual experiences that remain possible in living with dementia. These related to maintaining a positive self-concept but also focused both on the significance of other people as well as the 'bigger picture' beyond dementia. The literature base that related to this overarching theme and its three components may be nascent. However, it reflects an important gap in knowledge with regard to potentially significant aspects of people's experiences of living well with dementia. This therefore signposts an area for future clinical research on well-being in dementia.

A process of active life review appeared connected, in some studies, to a sense of gratitude to others and to a life well-lived, which, in turn, engendered a sense of satisfaction. The experience and function of gratitude in dementia has received little attention so far but it is a psychological factor known to be associated with positive physical health, positive emotion, life satisfaction and satisfying relationships (see Wood, Froh and Geraghty, 2010). In keeping with the notion that well-being in dementia is connected with positive selfhood (e.g. see Sabat, 2001) retaining a positive sense of self seems connected with a process of coming to accept dementia. An intriguing possibility relates to whether self-compassion – treating oneself with care, warmth and kindness in the face of adversity – could be involved in reaching acceptance (rather than resignation) whilst also upholding the experience of a stable and positive sense of identity as people live with dementia. Research work has started to highlight the significance of self-compassion for positive ageing (Allen and Leary, 2014) and it is therefore feasible to extend this approach to more fully understand what enables people to live well with dementia.

Perhaps controversially, the third component of this theme (*growing and transcending*) suggests that people with dementia might continue to experience aspects of personal and spiritual growth and that some people may have positive experiences not only in spite of the condition but, in certain ways, because of it. Literature in other areas highlights how living through traumatic or illness-related adversity can, for some, trigger a process of personal growth that can not only involve benefit finding as a way to maintain well-being but may also lead to a more fundamental and positive re-structuring of one's beliefs, values and relationships with others (Lechner, Tennen and Affleck, 2009). In Chapter 7, the potential for these types of experiences to shape the lives of people with dementia is explored.

POSITIVE EXPERIENCES IN DEMENTIA: THEMES, SUB-THEMES AND ILLUSTRATIVE QUOTES

1. ENGAGING WITH LIFE IN AGEING

a. *Seeking pleasure and enjoyment –
positive emotion in the here and now*

> 'I like the programmes where they ask questions and like that, to see if I can answer 'em…' ('Problem solving – engaging in activity'; Van Dijkhuizen, Clare and Pearce, 2006, p.87)

b. *Keeping going – persevering and feeling able*

> 'All the while I'm well enough to keep going, I'll keep going. And that's it.' ('I'm alright, I'll manage'; Clare *et al.*, 2008, p.716)

c. *Love and support – positive well-being through connections with others*

> 'I've got a good wife, you see; she's brilliant, she always helps me...a wonderful daughter and lots of good friends, you know – what more could I wish for really?' ('Always that connection versus it's not just me'; Caddell and Clare, 2011, p.392)

2. ENGAGING WITH DEMENTIA

a. *Facing it and fighting it – confronting, accepting and challenging dementia*

> 'Then you decide, well OK, we'll fight it as long as we can.' ('Developing a fighting spirit'; Clare, 2002, p.144)

b. *Humour – using laughter to diffuse dementia*

> 'I've got into the habit of making a joke about it; otherwise it would take over my life.' ('Normal versus abnormal memory loss – putting it into context'; Langdon, Eagle and Warner, 2007, p.995)

c. *Hope – a positive life force*

> 'If at first you don't succeed, there is no use giving up – if you don't hope for things, you don't get them.' ('Self activating hope'; Wolverson, Clarke and Moniz-Cook, 2010, p.454)

3. IDENTITY AND GROWTH

a. *Giving thanks – feeling and expressing gratitude and appreciation*

> 'I've had a tremendous life. I wouldn't trade it with anyone, and when it ends, you know, I'm just grateful for all I've had, and I'm hoping to enjoy every minute I've got left.' ('Life Review'; MacRae, 2010, p.300)

b. *Still being me – actively preserving a sense of self and self-worth*

> 'You've lost your memory but you haven't lost your mind. And you're still the same person.' ('Seeing self as the same person'; Werezak and Stewart, 2002, p.81)

c. *Growing and transcending – seeing beyond dementia to others and the spiritual realm*

> 'And what's lovely…people like me are retiring and getting Alzheimer's disease and all the rest, at home. All these other people are queuing up and waiting to go. So it's a big cycle.' ('Connections with people'; Dalby, Sperlinger and Boddington, 2011, p.89)

In conducting this review to determine positive experiences in older people who were living with dementia, we faced the challenge of synthesising positive findings from studies that had not originally focused explicitly on positive factors and experiences. Indeed, only 2 of the 26 included studies deliberately and explicitly explored positive factors and experiences in the lives of people with dementia. These were a study of *Hope* (Wolverson, Clarke and Moniz-Cook, 2010) and a study of *Spirituality* (Dalby, Sperlinger and Boddington, 2011). This highlights how previous clinical research has been subject to what can be termed a loss-deficit paradigm (described earlier), where meaningful positive experiences are assumed either to not exist or else only to represent a person's compensation against the negative effects of the condition.

POSITIVE PSYCHOLOGY AND DEMENTIA: CAVEATS AND OPPORTUNITIES

An important caveat to any findings relating to positive states and experiences in dementia concerns the so-called 'tyranny of the positives'. This important criticism has been levelled at the positive psychology movement itself (Held, 2004) and is a very real consideration in dementia. Oversimplified, the application of positive psychology to the experience of dementia risks conveying a message that positive experiences are easily achieved or that people simply need to think or act positively, whatever their circumstances, in order to live well.

Any such 'mandating' of positivity (Aspinwall and Tedeschi, 2010) also has the potential to attribute blame to a person if they find themselves unable to achieve a sense of living well.

Dementia poses profound and cumulative challenges to positive health and well-being, both directly (due to changes in cognitive and social abilities) and indirectly (through negative social positioning). To ignore this would be a profound disservice to those who attempt to live with and overcome these challenges. Thus, the search for a better understanding of aspects of positive experiences in dementia should never disallow people from the voicing of negative emotions and experiences or accessing support to alleviate them. A one-dimensional perspective on positive experiences in dementia would risk minimising the realities of the negative experiences people also have and this would move us away from a genuine person-centred approach.

Consistent with a 'second-wave' positive psychology perspective (e.g. see Lomas and Ivtzan, 2015), this book is therefore concerned with both the balance and meanings of positive *and* negative experiences in living with dementia and what these could mean in relation to living well. As with other chronic health conditions, negative and positive experiences and states in dementia could interact to determine personal meanings and responses. However, we cannot assume that positive experiences are ubiquitous in dementia or that they are easily or consistently experienced. We must also tread cautiously in assuming that positive psycho-social processes (e.g. acceptance, hope, love, etc.) automatically equate with positive outcomes in dementia (e.g. well-being and quality of life). Further research is needed to shed full light on these possibilities.

SUMMARY: A POSITIVE PERSON-CENTRED APPROACH TO DEMENTIA

The findings of our review (as described earlier and in Wolverson, Clarke and Moniz-Cook, 2016), indicate how positive experiences and attributes in dementia can co-occur and interact with negatives but nevertheless remain important aspects of personhood that must not be overlooked. The review's findings also provide empirical evidence for Kitwood's (1997) understanding of transcendence and his framework for well-being, where notions of love, identity, comfort and attachment are identified as important psychological needs for people with dementia. Kitwood's early work, set within an institutional context, became strongly associated with his Dementia Care Mapping observational system (Brooker and Surr, 2005), which has been used to systematically orient care practices towards positive interactions and therefore improve well-being in people with dementia living in care homes. There has been less study of the application of his theory of personhood for those who have to adjust to psychological threats to identity following an early diagnosis of dementia. Research into the strengths and positive experiences that people with dementia can themselves bring to these circumstances has been scarcer still.

If the central aim of a person-centred approach to dementia is to enable individuals to reach their well-being potential, then it is imperative that we fully understand people's 'optimal' experiences and particular personal strengths, as well as the social resources that underpin and maintain them. Accordingly, subsequent chapters in this book seek to develop our understanding of how people with dementia may flourish – that is, to live well and achieve an optimal level of functioning within the constraints posed by the condition. Aspects of Seligman's (2011) PERMA framework are highly pertinent to beginning to understand what flourishing could mean for people living with dementia, and these are also covered by particular chapters as follows:

> Positive emotions (hope: Chapter 4; humour: Chapter 5)

> Engagement (well-being: Chapter 3; creativity: Chapter 8)

> Relationships, where the quality of the relationship is key (relational dementia care: Chapter 10; positive aspects of caregiving: Chapter 11)

> Meaning, belonging to something greater than oneself (growth: Chapter 7; spirituality and wisdom: Chapter 9)

> Accomplishment, where persistence is an important quality (resilience: Chapter 6).

What particular processes underpin positive lived experiences and well-being in dementia? We may start to speculate that experiences of agency, flow, hopefulness, humour, intimacy, perseverance and transcendence are all important in process terms, and many of these issues are also explored in detail in the rest of this volume. Considering their role in dementia and the relationship they might have to well-being allows us to move towards a conceptual framework for the application of positive psychology to dementia research and care (see Chapter 12). However, this must also be a contextualised and balanced approach that incorporates the crucial influence the social environment has in supporting the expression and experience of personhood.

In summarising this chapter, it is therefore possible to highlight key connections between the person-centred approach to well-being in dementia and corresponding positive psychology constructs, whilst also drawing attention to aspects of positive social psychology (see Brooker, 2012) that are needed to foster well-being. An outline of what can be termed a *positive person-centered approach* to living well with dementia is thus summarised in Table 2.1 and this forms a reference framework for subsequent chapters of this book.

Table 2.1: Person-centred factors, corresponding positive psychology constructs and their potential relevance to living well with dementia

PERSON-CENTRED FACTORS	POSITIVE PSYCHOLOGY CONSTRUCTS	POTENTIAL FOR LIVING WELL
Identity and selfhood	Self-efficacy; self-compassion; personal growth in adversity; transcendence	People living with dementia can retain positive self-worth by feeling valued in their relationships and communities and by society. People can feel in control of personally important outcomes and retain or build the capacity for self-compassion in accepting a diagnosis of dementia. People can experience personal growth by finding new meanings in their experiences and/or continuing to age positively. Social environments need to support people to retain their sense of purpose and meaning as well as enabling self-compassion and personal growth.

cont.

PERSON-CENTRED FACTORS	POSITIVE PSYCHOLOGY CONSTRUCTS	POTENTIAL FOR LIVING WELL
Maintaining agency and autonomy	Hope, self-determination (balancing autonomy, competence and relatedness needs); personal strengths – courage and determination; optimism.	People can maintain a sense of themselves as the authors of their own decisions and actions. People can experience hope and optimism regarding the fulfilment of their own needs and the lives of loved ones. Social environments should support and meet needs for autonomy and competence whilst maintaining effective support and relatedness. Positive support should enable the capacity for courage and determination.
Social confidence; inclusion, belonging and reciprocity	Love; secure attachment; gratitude; altruism; forgiveness	People can maintain the capacity to give and receive love and kindness and express gratitude and forgiveness. Social environments need to promote inclusion in a way that enables these experiences and states – by emphasising belonging as well as providing opportunities for reciprocity.
Maintaining purpose and occupation	Flow; creativity; time perspective; hope	People can engage in purposeful and creative activities that offer personal meaning and a sense of competence in the here-and-now. Activities need to carry the potential for the optimal experiences through flow – a balance between perceived skills and perceived challenge that leads to absorption in an activity. Social environments should provide and support activities that enable these experiences to occur.
Emotional experience and expression	Positive emotions; humour; creativity; playfulness; positive reminiscence and life review	People can regularly experience pleasure, joy, serenity, laughter, humour, curiosity, interest and awe. Social environments must acknowledge these states as meaningful and enable their full expression.

In this chapter we have seen how a narrow, illness-focused construction of dementia has inadvertently fostered negative stereotypes and stigmatising social processes that have obscured our understanding of positive experiences and outcomes. However, social discourses surrounding dementia are now undergoing seismic changes, led by people living with it and sustained by concerted and international moves toward empowerment, inclusion and self-advocacy. In this new and evolving narrative, people living with dementia can be seen as active agents in their unfolding experience of the condition who, despite the formidable challenges they face, retain the capacity and motivation to increase their well-being and find ways to flourish. The chapters that follow explore and also demonstrate how this can be experienced.

REFERENCES

Allen, A.B. and Leary, M.R. (2014) 'Self-compassionate responses to aging.' *The Gerontologist 54*(2), 190–200.

Alzheimer's Disease International (2012) *World Alzheimer Report 2012.* Available at www.alz.co.uk, accessed on 15 April 2016.

Alzheimer's Society (2014) *Dementia 2014: Opportunity for Change.* Available at www.alzheimers.org.uk/dementia2014, accessed on 15 April 2016.

Aspinwall, L.G. and Tedeschi, R.G. (2010) 'The value of positive psychology for health psychology: Progress and pitfalls in examining the relation of positive phenomena to health.' *Annals of Behavioral Medicine 39*, 4–15.

Beard, R. (2004) 'In their voices: identity preservation and experiences of Alzheimer's disease.' *Journal of Aging Studies 18*, 415–428.

Behuniak, S.M. (2011) 'The living dead? The construction of people with Alzheimer's disease as zombies.'*Ageing and Society 31*(1), 70–92.

Brooker, D. (2012) 'Understanding dementia and the person behind the diagnostic label.' *International Journal of Person Centered Medicine 2*(1), 11–17.

Brooker D. and Surr C. (2005) *Dementia Care Mapping: Principles and Practice.* Bradford: Bradford Dementia Group.

Brunet, M.D., McCartney, M., Heath, I., Tomlinson, J. *et al.* (2012) 'There is no evidence base for proposed dementia screening.' *BMJ 345*, e8588.

Caddell, L.S. and Clare, L. (2011) 'I'm still the same person: The impact of early-stage dementia on identity.' *Dementia 10*(3) 379–398.

Clare, L. (2002) 'We'll fight it as long as we can: Coping with the onset of Alzheimer's disease.' *Aging and Mental Health 6*, 139–148.

Clare, L., Goater, T. and Woods, B. (2006) 'Illness representations in early-stage dementia: A preliminary investigation.' *International Journal of Geriatric Psychiatry 21*, 761–767.

Clare, L., Nelis, S.M., Quinn, C., Martyr, A. *et al.* (2014) 'Improving the experience of dementia and enhancing active life – living well with dementia: Study protocol for the IDEAL study.' *Health and Quality of Life Outcomes 12*, 164.

Clare, L., Roth, I. and Pratt, R. (2005) 'Perceptions of change over time in early-stage Alzheimer's Disease.' *Dementia 4*, 487–520.

Clare, L., Rowlands, J., Bruce, E., Surr, C. and Downs, M. (2008) '"I don't do like I used to do": A grounded theory approach to conceptualising awareness in people with moderate to severe dementia living in long-term care.' *Social Science and Medicine 66*(11), 2366–2377.

Dalby, P., Sperlinger, D. and Boddington, S. (2011) 'The lived experience of spirituality and dementia in older people living with mild to moderate dementia.' *Dementia 11*, 75–94.

de Boer, M., Hertogh, C., Droes, R., Riphagen, I., Jonker, C. and Eefsting, J. (2007) 'Suffering from dementia – the patient's perspective: A review of the literature.' *International Psychogeriatrics 19*, 1021–1039.

Deci, E.L. and Ryan, R.M. (2002) 'Overview of Self-determination Theory: An Organismic Dialectical Perspective.' In R.M. Ryan and E.L. Deci (eds) *Handbook of Self-determination Research*. Rochester, NY: The University of Rochester Press.

Department of Health (2009) *Living Well with Dementia: A National Dementia Strategy*. London: The Stationery Office.

Department of Health (2012) *Prime Minister's Challenge on Dementia – Delivering Major Improvements in Dementia Care and Research by 2015*. London: The Stationery Office.

Dewing, J. (2008) 'Personhood and dementia: Revisiting Tom Kitwood's ideas.' *International Journal of Older People Nursing 3*(1), 3–13.

Diehl, M., Hay, E.L. and Berg, K.M. (2011) 'The ratio between positive and negative affect and flourishing mental health across adulthood.' *Aging and Mental Health 15*(7), 882–893.

Dodge, R., Daly, A.P., Huyton, J. and Sanders, L.D. (2012) 'The challenge of defining well-being.' *International Journal of Well-being 2*(3), 222–235.

ESRO (2014) *A Good Life with Dementia*. London: ESRO. Available at www.esro.co.uk/publications, accessed on 19 July 2016.

Fredrickson, B.L. and Losada, M.F. (2005) 'Positive affect and the complex dynamics of human flourishing.' *American Psychologist 60*(7), 678–686.

George, D.R. and Whitehouse, P.J. (2014) 'The war (on terror) on Alzheimer's.' *Dementia 13*(1), 120–130.

Harman, G. and Clare, L. (2006) 'Illness representations and lived experience in early stage dementia.' *Qualitative Health Research 16*, 484–502.

Harris, P.B. and Keady, J. (2008) 'Wisdom, resilience and successful aging: Changing public discourses on living with dementia.' *Dementia 7*, 5–8.

Held, B.S. (2004) 'The negative side of positive psychology.' *Journal of Humanistic Psychology 44*, 9–46.

Kane, M. and Cook, L. (2013). *Dementia 2013: The Hidden Voice of Loneliness*. London: Alzheimer's Society.

Karran, E., Mercken, M. and De Strooper, B. (2011) 'The amyloid cascade hypothesis for Alzheimer's disease: An appraisal for the development of therapeutics.' *Nature Reviews Drug Discovery 10*(9), 698–712.

Kitwood, T. (1997) *Dementia Reconsidered*. Buckingham, MK: Open University Press.

Kitwood, T. and Bredin, K. (1992) 'Towards a theory of dementia care: Personhood and well-being.' *Ageing and Society 12*(3), 269–287.

Kolanowski, A.M., Litaker, M. and Buettner, L. (2005) 'Efficacy of theory-based activities for behavioural symptoms of dementia.' *Nursing Research 54*(4), 219–228.

Kontos, P. and Martin, W. (2013) 'Embodiment and dementia: Exploring critical narratives of selfhood, surveillance, and dementia care.' *Dementia 12*(3), 288–302.

Langdon, S.A., Eagle, A. and Warner, J. (2007) 'Making sense of dementia in the social world: A qualitative study.' *Social Science and Medicine 64*, 989–1000.

Lechner, S.C., Tennen, H. and Affleck, G. (2009) 'Benefit-finding and Growth.' In S.J. Lopez and C.R. Snyder (eds) *The Oxford Handbook of Positive Psychology*. New York: Oxford University Press.

Lomas, T. and Ivtzan, I. (2015) 'Second wave positive psychology: Exploring the positive–negative dialectics of well-being.' *Journal of Happiness Studies.* DOI: 10.1007/s10902-015-9668-y

MacRae, H. (2010) 'Managing identity while living with Alzheimer's Disease.' *Qualitative Health Research 20*(3), 293–305.

Maddux, J.E. (2009) 'Stopping the "Madness": Positive Psychology and Deconstructing the Illness Ideology and the DSM.' In S.J. Lopez and C.R. Snyder (eds) *The Oxford Handbook of Positive Psychology*. New York: Oxford University Press.

Mitchell, G.J., Dupuis, S.L. and Kontos, P. (2013) 'Dementia discourse: From imposed suffering to knowing other-wise.' *Journal of Applied Hermeneutics.* ISSN 1927-4416. Available at http://jah.journalhosting.ucalgary.ca/jah/index.php/jah/article/view/41, accessed on 15 April 2016.

Nakamura, J. and Csikszentmihalyi, M. (2009) 'Flow Theory and Research.' In S.J. Lopez and C.R.Snyder (eds) *The Oxford Handbook of Positive Psychology*. New York: Oxford University Press.

Paterson, B.L. (2001) 'The shifting perspectives model of chronic illness.' *Journal of Nursing Scholarship 33*(1), 21–26.

Peterson, C. and Seligman, M. (2004) *Character Strengths and Virtues: A Handbook and Classification*. New York, NY: Oxford University Press.

Poblador-Plou, B., Calderón-Larrañaga, A., Marta-Moreno, J., Hancco-Saavedra, J. *et al.* (2014) 'Comorbidity of dementia: A cross-sectional study of primary care older patients.' *BMC Psychiatry 14*(1), 84.

Portacolone, E., Berridge, C.K., Johnson, J. and Schicktanz, S. (2014) 'Time to reinvent the science of dementia: The need for care and social integration.' *Aging and Mental Health 18*(3), 269–275.

Post, S.G. (2013) 'Hope in caring for the deeply forgetful: Enduring selfhood and being open to surprises.' *Bulletin of the Menninger Clinic 77*(4), 349.

Rahman, S. (2014) *Living Well with Dementia: The Importance of the Person and the Environment for Well-being*. London: Radcliffe.

Rusk, R.D and Waters, L. (2014) 'A psycho-social system approach to well-being: Empirically deriving the Five Domains of Positive Functioning.' *The Journal of Positive Psychology 9*, 1–12.

Sabat, S.R. (2001) *The Experience of Alzheimer's Disease: Life Through a Tangled Veil.* Oxford: Blackwell.

Scholl, J.M. and Sabat, S.R. (2008) 'Stereotypes, stereotype threat and ageing: Implications for the understanding and treatment of people with Alzheimer's disease.' *Ageing and Society 28*(1), 103–130.

Seligman, M.E.P. (2011) *Flourish: A Visionary New Understanding of Happiness and Well-being.* New York, NY: Simon and Schuster.

Spector, A. and Orrell, M. (2010) 'Using a biopsychosocial model of dementia as a tool to guide clinical practice.' *International Psychogeriatrics 22*(6), 957–965.

Spector, A., Thorgrimsen, L., Woods, B.O.B., Royan, L. *et al.* (2003) 'Efficacy of an evidence-based cognitive stimulation therapy programme for people with dementia. Randomised controlled trial.' *The British Journal of Psychiatry 183*(3), 248–254.

Steeman, E., Godderis, J., Grypdonck, M., De Bal, N. and Dierckx De Casterle, B. (2007) 'Living with dementia from the perspective of older people: Is it a positive story?' *Aging and Mental Health 11*, 119–130.

Stirling, E. (2010) *Valuing Older People: Positive Psychological Practice.* Chichester: John Wiley and Sons.

Van Dijkhuizen, M., Clare, L. and Pearce, A. (2006) 'Striving for connection: Appraisal and coping among women with early-stage Alzheimer's disease.' *Dementia 5*, 73–94.

Wehmeyer, M.L., Little, T.D. and Sergeant, J. (2009) 'Self-Determination.' In S.J. Lopez and C.R. Snyder (eds) *The Oxford Handbook of Positive Psychology.* New York, NY: Oxford University Press.

Werezak, L. and Stewart, N. (2002) 'Learning to live with early dementia.' *The Canadian Journal of Nursing Research 34*, 67–85.

Whitehouse, P.J. and George, D. (2008) *The Myth of Alzheimer's: What You Aren't Being Told About Today's Most Dreaded Diagnosis.* New York, NY: St Martin's Press.

Wolverson, E., Clarke, C. and Moniz-Cook, E. (2010) 'Remaining hopeful in early-stage dementia: A qualitative study.' *Aging and Mental Health 14*(4), 450–460.

Wolverson, E.L., Clarke, C. and Moniz-Cook, E.D. (2016) 'Living positively with dementia: A systematic review and synthesis of the qualitative literature.' *Aging and Mental Health 20*(7), 676–699.

Wood, A.M., Froh, J.J. and Geraghty, A.W. (2010) 'Gratitude and well-being: A review and theoretical integration.' *Clinical Psychology Review 30*(7), 890–905.

World Health Organization (WHO) (2015) 'Governments commit to advancements in dementia research and care.' Available at www.who.int/mediacentre/news/releases/2015/action-on-dementia/en, accessed on 15 April 2016.

Wragg R.E. and Jeste D.V. (1989) 'Overview of depression and psychosis in Alzheimer's disease.' *American Journal of Psychiatry 146*(5), 577–587.

Chapter 3

WELL-BEING IN DEMENTIA

Alison Phinney

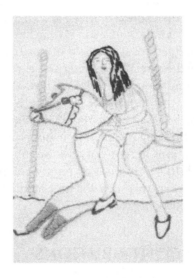

I recall my first semester as a doctoral student, sharing in class one day that I wanted to do research to understand what it was like to live with dementia. I had cared for people with dementia as a young hospital nurse and wanted to know what more could be done to support their quality of life. Specifically, I wanted to know what people with dementia experienced in their daily lives and what mattered to them. The professor – an esteemed scholar – agreed that this was a most interesting topic, but thought she should caution me that it was, of course, impossible to study. She believed, as did many others at that time, that there was no way to elicit the perspectives of people living with dementia. I persevered though, being lucky to find myself in a growing community of scholars who shared similar interests; and now, 20 years later, we have some understanding of the so-called 'subjective experience' of people with dementia.

Research that has explored this subjective perspective shows that living with dementia can be challenging, but, at the same time, the experience may not be as devastating as is often assumed. Hearing the voice of people with dementia has opened our eyes to the possibility of living well with dementia. People can, and do, report a good quality of life and are able to find meaning and experience satisfaction in their daily lives (e.g. Byrne-Davis, Bennett and Wilcock, 2006; Cahill *et al.*, 2004; Dröes *et al.*, 2006; Katsuno, 2005).

The purpose of this chapter is to explore the nature of well-being and quality of life in the context of living with dementia. To bring focus to the discussion, I begin by addressing some key perspectives on well-being that have emerged from the field of positive psychology and go on to consider how these relate to ageing and chronic illness in general. This serves as a foundation for exploring how these ideas might help further characterise the experience of living well with dementia. A critical examination of research on quality of life in dementia provides some direction in this regard but also exposes important conceptual and empirical limitations in terms of how the subjective experience has been handled. With this in mind, I go on to explore the growing body of qualitative inquiry in this area for its potential to inform a better understanding of well-being for people living with dementia.

WELL-BEING: CONTRIBUTIONS OF POSITIVE PSYCHOLOGY

Quality of life is an important and ubiquitous concept in the modern world, being understood and defined in a variety of ways and in a range of contexts. In particular, it holds a prominent place in the consideration of health, where it is generally viewed in terms of an individual's well-being in the context of daily living and especially in relation to their experience of illness. However, as a concept, quality of life is not without its limitations as it can be seen as lacking clear theoretical foundation whilst at the same time being widely held to encapsulate positive outcomes in health. Quality of life may be an important aspect of the broader concept of well-being, but there is a need to explore what other aspects of well-being could be of relevance to understanding living well with dementia. The field of positive psychology has made important contributions to understanding the idea of well-being, its subjective and psychological components, and its emotional aspects (see Chapter 1).

Broadly speaking, from a positive psychology perspective, well-being has been considered in two ways: 'Subjective well-being', typically represented in terms of happiness and life satisfaction, aligns with the so-called hedonic tradition, which equates well-being with positive emotional states like enjoyment and pleasure. 'Psychological well-being', on the other hand, is represented through ideas of human potential and flourishing, and aligns more closely with the eudemonic tradition that foregrounds such matters as personal growth, purpose and meaning in life. While subjective and psychological well-being are conceptually and empirically distinct, there are important connections between the two (Keyes, Shmotkin and Ryff, 2002) and it is likely that both are necessary components for a more comprehensive understanding of well-being (Henderson and Knight, 2012).

Diener (1984) argued that while there are objective conditions that influence quality of life, subjective well-being comes from an individual's perception of his or her own experience. Moreover, as an emotional evaluation, it is a complex accounting of *both* positive and negative emotions – it is not merely the absence of negative emotions. While some have made the specific argument that subjective well-being denotes a combination of low negative affect, high positive affect, and high life satisfaction (Diener *et al.*, 1999), the more general and important idea to come from this literature is that positive and negative affective states might co-occur and have distinct underlying processes and outcomes.

Drawing attention to the importance of positive feelings like joy, interest, contentment and love has been a particularly important contribution of the positive psychology field. Frederickson's 'broaden and build theory', for example, contends that while negative emotions such as fear and anger cause us to narrow our potential responses to situations, positive emotions open up possibilities for thought and action, which in turn contribute to building further intellectual, physical and social resources (Frederickson, 1998). In support, positive emotions have been shown to facilitate memory and information processing, and promote creative thinking. Positive emotions also contribute to social engagement by improving people's ability to offer and accept help from others. The ultimate benefit may be that positive emotions as a principal influence on subjective well-being are themselves protective of health and may even promote longevity (Diener and Chan, 2011).

As noted earlier, subjective well-being is not only how one feels in particular situations, but may also be framed in terms of life satisfaction, which is defined as the global evaluation one makes in considering one's life as a whole (Pavot and Diener, 2008). Repeated studies have shown that life satisfaction measured in this way tends to be quite stable; it varies little over time, even in the face of changing life circumstances. In part, this may be due to the fact that it correlates highly with stable personality traits like extraversion or neuroticism. It may also be the result of adaptation, whereby people are able to adjust to changes in their lives, thus maintaining consistency in how they evaluate their life satisfaction. That said, there are significant life events, such as the onset of disability or the loss of a spouse, that may have lasting impact on how people evaluate their satisfaction with their life as a whole (Pavot and Diener, 2008).

Coming from the perspective of subjective well-being, life satisfaction is considered to be an evaluation of the extent to which one is living a happy life. This is distinct from the concept of psychological well-being, which prioritises the goal of living a meaningful life. Carol Ryff's work in this area has been very influential. Drawing inspiration from the field of humanistic psychology, she posited that there are six universal needs – self-acceptance, positive relationships, autonomy, environmental mastery, purpose in life and personal growth – and argued that psychological well-being derives from the degree to which these various needs are met (Ryff, 1989a). Viewed in this way, well-being has an enduring quality as a relatively stable interpretation of how one is living up to the things that matter in one's life, reflecting the sense that one's life is meaningful. This perspective may be particularly important for understanding the potential for well-being in the context of life challenges such as those experienced in advanced age and illness.

WELL-BEING IN AGEING AND CHRONIC ILLNESS

Research has consistently indicated that well-being does not always diminish with age and that different aspects of well-being have different trajectories in later life. For example, negative affect seems to stay stable while life satisfaction may even increase (Charles, Reynolds and Gatz, 2001). Overall, it seems that older people tend to maintain a fairly optimistic view of their lives. Carol Ryff (1989b) asked 102 older people about their well-being and what it meant to them. Most reported themselves to be happy and satisfied with their current circumstances and were not interested in changing anything in their lives. As to their psychological well-being, a majority reported that the most important feature was having positive and caring relationships with others. The importance of social and relational factors has since been confirmed through a meta-analysis of over 200 studies showing that the quality of social contacts is strongly associated with subjective well-being among older adults (Pinquart and Sorenson, 2000).

Research has also shown that involvement in activity is a key factor supporting well-being in ageing. Recent systematic reviews have confirmed that exercise significantly improves the mood and psychological well-being of older people (e.g. see Windle *et al.*, 2010). An extensive critical review of 42 studies exploring the benefits of activity for older people found that a majority of the studies reported a positive relationship between participation in activity and psychological well-being, with informal social and leisure activity seeming to have the most influence (Adams, Leibbrandt and Moon, 2011). Building on the results of their review, these authors further argued that having a *choice* about which activities to engage in, and the *perceived value* and *meaning* of the activities, are likely to be the most important mediating factors in this relationship, although they noted that further research was required.

There have been numerous attempts to theorise what it means to 'age well'. Rowe and Kahn's model of 'Successful Ageing' (see Rowe and Kahn, 1997) posits that so-called successful ageing comprises three components: 'low probability of disease and disease-related disability; high cognitive and physical functional capacity; and active engagement with life' (p.433). The authors define active engagement in terms of social relationships and productive activity, which, as we have seen in the more recent empirical evidence, are closely related to subjective well-being. This model of Successful Ageing has not been without its detractors, however, particularly in light of the fact that a majority of older people will live with one or more chronic health conditions that limit their functional capacity and cause some degree of disability.

A normative model that excludes so many would seem to be of limited value (Martinson and Berridge, 2015). Strawbridge, Wallhagen and Cohen (2002) made this point clearly when they analysed data from a large longitudinal study of ageing to find that 43 per cent of older people with one chronic condition and 35 per cent of those with two chronic conditions identified themselves as 'ageing successfully', a result that the Rowe and Kahn model could not account for.

Subjective approaches to the study of successful ageing may extend our understanding of this phenomenon. A recent systematic review found that studies using self-ratings of successful ageing showed a much higher prevalence than those using objective researcher-defined ratings; far more people identify themselves as ageing well than would be predicted using objective criteria alone (Cosco et al., 2014). While the overall number of studies remains small, these kinds of results point to the idea that positive experiences of ageing are achievable even for those who face significant adversity due to illness. Subjective measures are often critiqued for being prone to 'bias', but what this fails to recognise is their potential to reveal the complexity and contextual richness that contributes to these kinds of evaluations. People's experiences of ageing do not lend themselves to a simple 'either-or' calculation; living well with chronic illness is a complicated question demanding a more holistic approach that includes subjective components (Cosco et al., 2014).

WELL-BEING AND QUALITY OF LIFE IN DEMENTIA

Over the last 15 years there has been a growing body of literature examining the even more complicated question of what it might mean to live well and experience positive well-being with dementia. The earliest conceptual work in this area emerged in the early 1990s, with two scholars being particularly influential. Powell Lawton in the USA used the terminology of 'quality of life' (which has been commonly used in the field of gerontology) and drew attention to both its subjective and objective dimensions. He argued that while quality of life could be observed and evaluated by others according to normative criteria, it was also important to consider people's self-evaluations (Lawton, 1994). At the same time in the UK, Tom Kitwood was seeking to improve quality of care in order to enhance the 'well-being' of people with dementia, which he argued should be *the* guiding concern of all care providers. He conceptualised well-being in relational terms, bringing the language of *personhood* into the caring lexicon (see Chapter 2).

This early conceptual work was followed soon after by innovations in measurement. At the same time that Lawton and Kitwood were putting the person with dementia in the foreground and articulating ground-breaking ideas about quality of life and well-being in dementia, the first drug treatment trials were starting. While manufacturers were at that time mostly focused on the impact of treatment on cognition, mood, behaviour and caregiver burden, the idea that something could be done for people with dementia to improve their lives helped bolster interest in the scientific community to consider quality of life as a potentially important outcome. With a growing subject pool of people with earlier-stage dementia being solicited for these drug trials, researchers were prompted to consider the idea that people with dementia could report on their own quality of life, at least in the early stages of the disease. Given this context, the earliest research on quality of life and well-being in dementia was focused on how it could be assessed or measured.

APPROACHES TO MEASUREMENT

To date, there have been at least 16 different instruments developed to measure quality of life in dementia (Bowling *et al.*, 2015). These reflect a range of conceptual underpinnings and are in varying formats, with most relying on some form of proxy report. Only a few have aimed to evaluate the experience of the person with dementia, either through self-report or observation.

Of these, the Dementia Quality of Life (D-QoL) tool was the first to be published (Brod *et al.*, 1999), and remains one of the only measures that relies exclusively on the self-report of people with dementia (the other being the Bath Assessment of Subjective Quality of Life in Dementia (BASQID; Trigg *et al.*, 2007), which has had limited application). Brod *et al.* (1999) conducted focus groups with community-dwelling people with mild to moderate dementia, caregivers and expert clinicians, and from this developed a 29-item self-report measure. The tool has five domains: self-esteem, positive affect, negative affect, aesthetics and feelings of belonging. In contrast, the Quality of Life–Alzheimer's Disease scale (QoL-AD), developed by Logsdon and colleagues (1999), comprises 13 items that were developed on the basis of a literature review, and were subsequently reviewed by older people with and without dementia and a panel of clinicians and researchers experienced in the field. The tool covers a range of concepts, including physical, mental and cognitive health, social situation, functional ability and life as a whole. It exists in both self-report and proxy format, and yields a single overall score.

These two instruments have been widely used in research, primarily with community populations of people with mild to moderate dementia. Measuring quality of life for those with more advanced disease remains a challenge. Observational tools have been conceptualised as a way to get closer to the experience of the person without having to rely on self-report. Dementia Care Mapping (DCM) is the most widely recognised of these (Brooker, 2005). Based on Kitwood's conceptualisation of well-being and personhood (1997), DCM uses a coding scheme to systematically identify and evaluate people's experiences of well-being or ill-being. It was developed as a practice tool to demonstrate to carers the nature of their interactions and the effect this can have on a person's well-being. As a research instrument, it is lengthy and requires a significant time commitment, which may explain why it has been used in only a small number of published studies.

FACTORS INFLUENCING RATINGS OF QUALITY OF LIFE IN DEMENTIA

In the last 10 years, there has been a growing body of research into the factors that influence quality of life in dementia. Banerjee *et al.* (2009) conducted a comprehensive review to explore this question, relying as much as possible on research using self-report measures. They found the research to be quite variable, not only in terms of how quality of life had been defined and measured, but also as regards the participants studied and their respective settings. Nevertheless, there do seem to be two factors that are consistently related to quality of life.

The first factor is who is doing the assessment. Research has shown repeatedly that proxy measures are almost always lower than self-report. People living with dementia perceive their quality of life more positively than do their caregivers, possibly because proxy ratings are unduly influenced by low well-being in the caregiver (Schultz *et al.*, 2013). The second factor is depression. People living with dementia who are depressed are more likely to report lower quality of life, at least in the mild to moderate stages of the illness. The direction of the causal relationship is unclear, however, and there remains a need for further research to help us understand whether depression causes poor quality of life, or if poor quality of life causes depression.

Just as important are the factors that are unrelated to quality of life. While memory complaints may impact quality of life in older people without dementia (Mol *et al.*, 2007), this relationship seems to be different for those living with dementia. Research has repeatedly shown that a person's level of cognitive impairment seems to have little consistent bearing on their self-reported quality of life. The picture is somewhat less clear when considering the effect of functional impairment. People's ability to engage in everyday activities may have an effect on how they rate their quality of life, but the research findings have been somewhat mixed.

The take-home message here seems to be that the factors we might expect to be important are experienced quite differently by people living with dementia themselves, who tend to rate their quality of life quite highly. Cognitive and functional decline do not seem to have a significant impact on subjective reports of quality of life, and (at least in the mild to moderate stages of the illness) there appear to be important similarities between people with dementia and those without in terms of how they experience and interpret their own well-being.

But even with these similarities, dementia is likely to remain an important fact in people's lives. Many people will be living with very real challenges. It is better perhaps to interpret the existing research as showing that quality of life in dementia is complex and multi-dimensional, and as such is not easily broken down into measurement scales and simple research designs. Despite the growing volume of work being conducted in this area, really very little is currently understood (Venturato, 2010). Most of the research has centred on the development and use of measurement tools, which arguably have limited validity. They have been under-theorised, and moreover, by their very designs are not sensitive to the moment-by-moment experiences of well-being that may be most important for people living with dementia.

Here is where qualitative research exploring the subjective experiences of people with dementia may contribute to a more complete and contextualised understanding of what it means to live well. An example is seen in the research by Steeman and colleagues, who conducted a grounded theory study to understand how people with early-stage dementia evaluate their lives (Steeman *et al.*, 2007).

Their preliminary analysis suggested a positive storyline that minimised problems and emphasised people's contentment with their lives. But by taking their analysis deeper, they identified a more complex experience of people with dementia trying to achieve a 'balance' between feeling valued and feeling worthless. However, one might argue that these negative and positive experiences are not opposite ends of a continuum – as the balance metaphor might suggest – but rather they exist in tandem, with both being important dimensions of living with dementia.

This kind of finding warrants a closer look at the qualitative research being conducted in this area. In the last 20 years there has been a growing body of research seeking to understand the lived experiences of people with dementia, again focused largely on those in the mild to moderate stages. While little of this has directly addressed the question of well-being, many of the findings inform an understanding of this important concept.

LIVED EXPERIENCES

In the discussion that follows, I explore what seem to be three important aspects of well-being (selfhood and identity; purpose and belonging; and meaning and pleasure) as expressed by people living with dementia (see the various 'Experiences' below), and via existing lived experience research. The purpose here is to better understand the lived experience of well-being in dementia and the conditions under which it can be nurtured and sustained.

Experiences of well-being – life is good!

Maggie was my first study participant. She was 70, and a year previously had been forced to retire when it became increasingly difficult for her to manage the demands of her work. From the time we spent together I could see that everyday life was hard for her. Activities she had previously taken for granted took a lot of effort and increasingly she was relying on her husband to look after the household. Her days were simple. She spent much of her time alone, sometimes going out for a walk in the nearby park, asking strangers for directions when she was not sure which way to turn. It was hard for Maggie to express herself, and she often seemed frustrated in our conversations together. So it surprised me one day that when I asked her the difficult question of what she saw ahead for herself, she burst out saying 'Oh, I want to live to be 100!' Smiling and energised, she went on tell me about how her life was good and she wanted it to continue just as it was. I understood that she was not putting me off; this was not a superficial answer borne of denial. Maggie recognised that her life was not easy, but she continued to see possibilities for joy and contentment. She had a feeling of connection in her world, and she knew that her life mattered. Her words were an expression of a quite profound sense of well-being. They have stayed with me for many years.

---

1. SELFHOOD AND IDENTITY

Dementia can pose a profound threat to a person's sense of self. The stigma associated with a dementia diagnosis and resulting experiences of discrimination, whereby people are discounted and excluded from the world around them can have a significant impact on a person's self-esteem. '[When] they know you have Alzheimer's, they...leave you alone because they figure you don't know what you're talking about, you don't know what is going on. Oh, I used to hate that' (Katsuno, 2005, p.206).

In response, people living with dementia want to feel 'normal' and accepted by others and to be treated as they always were (Langdon, Eagle and Warner, 2007; von Kutzleben *et al.*, 2012). Staying active and engaged in life, and downplaying any problems encountered, are all ways people find to preserve a positive sense of self (De Boer *et al.*, 2007). This is further supported by being included and treated with respect by those around them. '[It is important] that people are kind and cheerful to me, as I am' (Droes *et al.*, 2006, p.541).

Continuity is an important theme in people's lives when faced with the challenges of dementia (Page and Keady, 2010). A metasynthesis of 33 qualitative studies showed the depth of people's resilience reflected in the range of strategies that are adopted in the interest of 'self-protection' (Steeman *et al.*, 2006). Feeling identity to be essentially unchanged, despite changing circumstances, is an important aspect of well-being for people living with dementia.

Experiences of well-being – the 'inner me'

Tom was a retired teacher and skilled carpenter who had designed and built the family home. He continued to embody that role, taking great delight in overseeing the construction of a wall on his property, and teaching me how to swing an adze. 'I'm in the old habit of being a schoolteacher and watching what everybody does', he said. This allowed him to feel that there was something about him that his Alzheimer's would never touch: 'I just have an inner me that isn't affected by it.'

2. PURPOSE AND BELONGING

Being able to live with a sense of purpose is important for the well-being of people with dementia (Droes *et al.*, 2006). Recognising that abilities may be failing or that one has an increasing need for help does not detract from an ongoing desire to be connected and of service to others (van der Roest *et al.*, 2007).

In part, feeling a sense of purpose is about being able to engage in activities that are oriented towards a particular goal (see 'Experiences... feeling useful'). Mak (2010) reported the results of an experimental study showing that people with dementia who drew a greeting card for a sick child or a soldier serving abroad reported higher levels of life purpose than those who made a similar drawing but with no specific goal in mind. This example draws attention to the important point that the purpose needs to be one that is socially significant, such that the activity provides a sense of belonging and connection with others. People with dementia often interpret their well-being in terms of the social interactions and emotional attachments they have with their families and communities (Byrne-Davis *et al.*, 2006; Cahill and Diaz-Ponce, 2011). These relationships go both ways: people certainly value the love and support they receive from their families but being able to contribute in worthwhile ways to the lives of others is just as important to people's well-being (Moyle *et al.*, 2010).

Experiences of well-being – feeling useful

Bebe was lost and ill at ease in her own home, pacing back and forth, disoriented and lamenting that there was nothing for her to do. This stood in marked contrast to her experience at the day programme, where she was encouraged to take part in preparing sandwiches and serving meals to the other group members. Being allowed to feel useful made a profound difference to Bebe's well-being. I watched as her entire demeanour changed; she moved with confidence, smiling as she looked around the common room saying 'home sweet home'.

---

3. MEANING AND PLEASURE

The question of meaning in the experiences of people living with dementia has been addressed in only a few studies (e.g. McFadden, Ingram and Baldauf, 2001; Menne, Kinney and Morhardt, 2002; Phinney, 2011; Phinney, Chaudhury and O'Connor, 2007) but would seem to be critical in understanding well-being. Most of the subjective experience literature focuses on loss and suffering, emphasising all that is negative as if no other kind of experience exists. This singular focus does a disservice to the complexity of the lives of people with dementia, perhaps reflecting more the fixation of researchers on delineating what is wrong so solutions can be targeted. However, looking more carefully, threaded throughout these research reports we see evidence of how people experience a wide range of emotions, and in particular, how they retain the capacity for joy and delight (see 'Experiences of well-being – "music is a blessing"'). Quality of life is enhanced when people have the opportunity to enjoy pleasurable activities, experience positive feelings and have fun (Cahill and Diaz-Ponce, 2011; Droes, 2006).

Experiences of well-being – 'music is a blessing'

Don was a retired priest who had for many years sung in an amateur choir. Music remained to him a deeply meaningful pastime. He explained it thus: '[Music] fills up my interest, my activities, my time, my desire... To put it very bluntly, music is a blessing, a blessing that I can express joy and happiness and all the good things that come with it, and fun.' Music continues to matter deeply to Don, even though he is no longer able to keep up with the demands of choral singing. Instead, his friend comes by his home once a week and sits down at the piano to play some of his favourite hymns. He takes this as an invitation to sit beside her and join her in song.

Emotional experiences like these are not merely passive reactions to positive stimuli, but rather they reflect how people are meaningfully engaged in a situation. This meaningful engagement happens when people are afforded the freedom to make choices that allow them to live up to personal values (McFadden *et al.*, 2001). Sometimes these are small opportunities, and sometimes they are big. This freedom to choose can be a challenge for people living with dementia and they may need added support for these meaningful moments.

PROGRAMMES AND INTERVENTIONS

Having discussed how to better understand and evaluate well-being and quality of life in dementia, a critical question remains: What can be done to improve it? So-called 'non-pharmacological interventions' tend to take a medicalised view of dementia, having as their goal improved function or cognition, or reduction of 'behavioural and psychological symptoms' (e.g. agitation, depression or wandering). Well-being and quality of life, if they are considered at all, are only a secondary concern. But as we have seen, there is growing interest in a personhood perspective that foregrounds subjective experience and envisions possibilities for meaning. This approach supports the development of interventions with potential for improving the well-being and quality of life of people living with dementia, potentially with respect to the core themes described.

Reminiscence and life story work have been a focus of considerable interest for many years in practice and research. Numerous studies have shown that these kinds of activities can be effective in creating moments of pleasure and enjoyment for people with dementia and may support their interactions with each other (Moos and Björn, 2006), although the quality of this evidence is not yet strong. Even now, there remains considerable variability in the design of the interventions and programmes themselves, and their effect on quality of life tends to be defined quite broadly.

Music and creative expression are drawing increased attention, given their obvious potential to support the well-being of people living with dementia. This is an area of practice that is developing rapidly and encompasses a broad array of *participatory* arts (as distinct from therapeutic forms), including music, dance, visual art, poetry and theatre (Zeilig, Killick and Fox, 2014). A growing body of literature supports the claim that these kinds of programmes and interventions are beneficial for people with dementia, although relatively few studies have directly addressed their impact on quality of life and subjective well-being (Beard, 2011). However, there are traces of evidence to suggest that involvement in creative activity can play a role in improving quality of life for people with dementia (Fraser, Bungay and Munn-Giddings, 2014). This may be through fostering a sense of belonging and being valued (Camic, Tischler and Pearman, 2014), or by enhancing social connections and feelings of happiness and pleasure (Sixsmith and Gibson, 2007).

Exercise appears to have numerous benefits for people living with dementia, with a number of studies showing improved mobility and slower rates of functional decline (Pitkälä *et al.*, 2013). Fewer studies have investigated outcomes of quality of life and subjective well-being, but results suggest that these too can be improved through exercise interventions (Potter *et al.*, 2011), possibly because it can be a meaningful activity for people with dementia. Cedervall and Åberg (2014), in an interview study of 14 people with mild dementia, found that physical activity provided for them a sense of normality and continuity, which enhanced their feelings of well-being and supported their sense of selfhood. Similarly, our own research has shown that people with mild to moderate dementia find walking to be a particularly meaningful activity; in part 'it's just something you do – you walk all your life' – and because walking with others provided valued companionship (McDuff and Phinney, 2015).

Social activity is recognised as a key opportunity for supporting well-being and quality of life in dementia. People with dementia who take part in daycare programmes and leisure activity groups have emphasised the importance of the social relationships they form with other members, relationships that in turn enhance their well-being (Brataas *et al.*, 2010; Dabelko-Schoeny and King, 2010). Support groups also benefit members through the social relationships they engender and the peer support that is offered (Dow *et al.*, 2011; Logsdon, 2010). These kinds of programmes and groups are thought to provide emotionally safe environments for people with dementia that allow them to feel understood and accepted (Phinney and Moody, 2011; Wiersma and Pedlar, 2008).

It is worth noting that social activities that are capable of enhancing well-being need not be extended experiences. Nor are they necessarily captured by general ratings of quality of life. Pringle (2003) offered the compelling argument that people with dementia can be supported to live 'rich, interesting, and pleasurable lives', and that what matters is the 'quality of the moment' (p.9). Recent research has shown support for this claim. McGilton and colleagues (McGilton *et al.*, 2012) studied brief interactions between care providers and residents with dementia, and found that the quality of these interactions directly influenced residents' emotional experiences. In this way, they showed that 'relating well does matter' (p.514), even in the fleeting moments of everyday activity.

CONCLUSIONS

Over the last 15 years there have been an increasing number of studies calling for greater attention to the perspectives and experiences of older people with chronic conditions, offering the argument that by including these 'missing voices' (Martinson and Berridge, 2015) we will be afforded a richer, more inclusive picture of what it means to age well. This is especially the case for those living with dementia. While much of the research reflects a persistent preference for a medicalised view of dementia, there is growing interest in person-centred outcomes focusing on positive psychology concepts. This chapter has examined emerging evidence from two broad areas of inquiry: quantitative research measuring quality of life in dementia and identifying its determinants, and qualitative research exploring the subjective experiences of well-being of people with dementia. From this, we can start to see how people living with dementia are active agents with the potential to experience quality of life and well-being. Certainly, dementia comes with inevitable challenges, but at the same time people can continue to find their lives meaningful and worth living, and welcome experiences of joy and contentment.

This idea brings to the foreground some important implications. Researchers, practitioners and policy makers need to agree that quality of life and well-being outcomes are not matters of secondary interest to be considered only after problems of function and behaviour have been addressed. There is no shortage of good ideas for programmes and interventions that provide meaning and enjoyment for people with dementia, support their sense of self and continuity and enrich their social connections. These experiences exist at the core of what it means to be human and an active and engaged citizen. More needs to be done to support the development and implementation of such programmes and interventions for people living with dementia both within the healthcare sector and more broadly in the community at large. Individual and social differences almost certainly have an important impact on people's experiences of well-being and quality of life in dementia. Understanding these differences will allow interventions and programmes to be better tailored to meet particular needs. This requires further research to determine what works, for whom, and in which contexts. Moreover, it is timely to be recognising the potential contributions of positive psychology to this important work. Interdisciplinary innovation that draws concepts of well-being together with emerging insights from the health and social gerontology fields will provide a foundation for the development of approaches to care and support that are most meaningful for people with dementia themselves.

REFERENCES

Adams, K.B., Leibbrandt, S. and Moon, H. (2011) 'A critical review of the literature on social and leisure activity and wellbeing in later life.' *Ageing and Society 31*(4), 683–712.

Banerjee, S., Samsi, K., Petrie, C.D., Alvir, J. et al. (2009) 'What do we know about quality of life in dementia? A review of the emerging evidence on the predictive and explanatory value of disease specific measures of health related quality of life in people with dementia.' *International Journal of Geriatric Psychiatry* 24(1), 15–24.

Beard, R.L. (2011) 'Art therapies and dementia care: A systematic review.' *Dementia* 11(5) 633–656.

Bowling, A., Rowe, G., Adams, S., Sands, P. et al. (2015) 'Quality of life in dementia: A systematically conducted narrative review of dementia-specific measurement scales.' *Ageing and Mental Health* 19(1), 13–31.

Brataas, H.V., Bjugan, H., Wille, T. and Hellzen, O. (2010) 'Experiences of day care and collaboration among people with mild dementia.' *Journal of Clinical Nursing* 19(19–20), 2839–2848.

Brod, M., Stewart, A.L., Sands, L. and Walton, P. (1999) 'Conceptualization and measurement of quality of life in dementia: The dementia quality of life instrument (DQoL).' *The Gerontologist* 39(1), 25–36.

Brooker, D. (2005) 'Dementia care mapping: A review of the research literature.' *The Gerontologist* 45(1), 11–18.

Byrne-Davis, L.M.T., Bennett, P.D. and Wilcock, G.K. (2006) 'How are quality of life ratings made? Toward a model of quality of life in people with dementia.' *Quality of Life Research* 15(5), 855–865.

Cahill, S., Begley, E., Topo, P., Saarikalle, K. et al. (2004) '"I know where this is going and I know it won't go back": Hearing the individual's voice in dementia quality of life assessments.' *Dementia* 3(3), 313–330.

Cahill, S. and Diaz-Ponce, A.M. (2011) '"I hate having nobody here. I'd like to know where they all are": Can qualitative research detect differences in quality of life among nursing home residents with different levels of cognitive impairment?' *Ageing and Mental Health* 15(5), 562–572.

Camic, P.M., Tischler, V. and Pearman, C.H. (2014) 'Viewing and making art together: A multi-session art-gallery-based intervention for people with dementia and their carers.' *Ageing and Mental Health* 18(2), 161–168.

Cedervall, Y. and Åberg, A.C. (2010) 'Physical activity and implications on well-being in mild Alzheimer's disease: A qualitative case study on two men with dementia and their spouses.' *Physiotherapy Theory and Practice* 26(4), 226–239.

Charles, S.T., Reynolds, C.A. and Gatz, M. (2001) 'Age-related differences and change in positive and negative affect over 23 years.' *Journal of Personality and Social Psychology* 80(1), 136–151.

Cosco, T.D., Prina, A.M., Perales, J., Stephan, B. and Brayne, C. (2014) 'Operational definitions of successful ageing: A systematic review.' *International Psychogeriatrics* 26(3), 373–381.

Dabelko-Schoeny, H. and King, S. (2010) 'In their own words: Participants' perceptions of the impact of adult day services.' *Journal of Gerontological Social Work* 53(2), 176–192.

De Boer, M.E., Hertogh, C.M., Dröes, R.M., Riphagen, I.I., Jonker, C. and Eefsting, J.A. (2007) 'Suffering from dementia – the patient's perspective: A review of the literature.' *International Psychogeriatrics* 19(6), 1021–1039.

Diener, E. (1984) 'Subjective well-being.' *Psychological Bulletin* 95, 542–575.

Diener, E. and Chan, M.Y. (2011) 'Happy people live longer: Subjective well-being contributes to health and longevity.' *Applied Psychology: Health and Well-Being* 3(1), 1–43.

Diener, E., Suh, E.M., Lucas, R.E. and Smith, H.L. (1999) 'Subjective well-being: Three decades of progress.' *Psychological Bulletin 125*, 276–302.

Dow, B., Haralambous, B., Hempton, C., Hunt, S. and Calleja, D. (2011) 'Evaluation of Alzheimer's Australia Vic Memory Lane Cafés.' *International Psychogeriatrics 23*, 246–255.

Dröes, R.M., Boelens-Van Der Knoop, E.C., Bos, J., Meihuizen, L. *et al.* (2006) 'Quality of life in dementia in perspective: An explorative study of variations in opinions among people with dementia and their professional caregivers, and in literature.' *Dementia 5*(4), 533–558.

Fraser, A., Bungay, H. and Munn-Giddings, C. (2014) 'The value of the use of participatory arts activities in residential care settings to enhance the well-being and quality of life of older people: A rapid review of the literature.' *Arts and Health* 6(3), 266–278.

Fredrickson, B.L. (1998) 'What good are positive emotions?' *Review of General Psychology 2*(3), 300–319.

Henderson, L.W. and Knight, T. (2012) 'Integrating the hedonic and eudaimonic perspectives to more comprehensively understand wellbeing and pathways to wellbeing.' *International Journal of Wellbeing 2*(3), 196–221.

Katsuno, T. (2005) 'Dementia from the inside: How people with early-stage dementia evaluate their quality of life.' *Ageing and Society 25*(2), 197–214.

Keyes, C.L., Shmotkin, D. and Ryff, C.D. (2002) 'Optimizing well-being: The empirical encounter of two traditions.' *Journal of Personality and Social Psychology 82*(6), 1007–1022.

Kitwood, T. (1997) *Dementia Reconsidered*. Buckingham: Open University Press.

Langdon, S.A., Eagle, A. and Warner, J. (2007) 'Making sense of dementia in the social world: A qualitative study.' *Social Science and Medicine 64*(4), 989–1000.

Lawton, M.P. (1994) 'Quality of life in Alzheimer disease.' *Alzheimer Disease and Associated Disorders 8*, 138–150.

Logsdon, R.G., Gibbons, L.E., McCurry, S.M. and Teri, L. (1999) 'Quality of life in Alzheimer's disease: Patient and caregiver reports.' *Journal of Mental Health and Ageing 5*, 21–32.

Logsdon, R.G., Pike, K.C., McCurry, S.M., Hunter, P. *et al.* (2010) 'Early-stage memory loss support groups: Outcomes from a randomized controlled clinical trial.' *Journals of Gerontology, Series B: Psychological Sciences and Social Sciences 65B*, 691–697.

Mak, W. (2010) 'Self-reported goal pursuit and purpose in life among people with dementia.' *The Journals of Gerontology Series B: Psychological Sciences and Social Sciences 66B*(2), 177–184.

Martinson, M. and Berridge, C. (2015) 'Successful ageing and its discontents: A systematic review of the social gerontology literature.' *The Gerontologist 55*, 58–69.

McDuff, J. and Phinney, A. (2015) 'Walking with meaning: Subjective experiences of physical activity in dementia.' *International Journal of Qualitative Nursing Research* 2. DOI: 2333393615605116

McFadden, S.H., Ingram, M. and Baldauf, C. (2001) 'Actions, feelings, and values: Foundations of meaning and personhood in dementia.' *Journal of Religious Gerontology 11*(3–4), 67–86.

McGilton, K.S., Sidani, S., Boscart, V.M., Guruge, S. and Brown, M. (2012) 'The relationship between care providers' relational behaviors and residents' mood and behavior in long-term care settings.' *Ageing and Mental Health 16*(4), 507–515.

Menne, H.L., Kinney, J.M. and Morhardt, D.J. (2002) 'Trying to continue to do as much as they can do: Theoretical insights regarding continuity and meaning making in the face of dementia.' *Dementia 1*(3), 367–382.

Mol, M., Carpay, M., Ramakers, I., Rozendaal, N., Verhey, F. and Jolles, J. (2007) 'The effect of perceived forgetfulness on quality of life in older adults: A qualitative review.' *International Journal of Geriatric Psychiatry 22*(5), 393–400.

Moos, I. and Björn, A. (2006) 'Use of the life story in the institutional care of people with dementia: A review of intervention studies.' *Ageing and Society 26*(3), 431–454.

Moyle, W., Venturto, L., Griffiths, S., Grimbeek, P. *et al.* (2011) 'Factors influencing quality of life for people with dementia: A qualitative perspective.' *Ageing and Mental Health 15*(8), 970–977.

Page, S. and Keady, J. (2010) 'Sharing stories: A meta-ethnographic analysis of 12 autobiographies written by people with dementia between 1989 and 2007.' *Ageing and Society 30*(3), 511–526.

Pavot, W. and Diener, E. (2008) 'The satisfaction with life scale and the emerging construct of life satisfaction.' *The Journal of Positive Psychology 3*(2), 137–152.

Phinney, A. (2011) 'Horizons of meaning in dementia: Retained and shifting narratives.' *Journal of Religion, Spirituality and Ageing 23*(3), 254–268.

Phinney, A., Chaudhury, H. and O'Connor, D.L. (2007) 'Doing as much as I can do: The meaning of activity for people with dementia.' *Ageing and Mental Health 11*(4), 384–393.

Phinney, A. and Moody, E.M. (2011) 'Leisure connections: benefits and challenges of participating in a social recreation group for people with early dementia.' *Activities, Adaptation and Ageing 35*(2), 111–130.

Pinquart, M. and Sörensen, S. (2000) 'Influences of socioeconomic status, social network, and competence on subjective well-being in later life: A meta-analysis.' *Psychology and Ageing 15*(2), 187–224.

Pitkälä, K., Savikko, N., Poysti, M., Strandberg, T. and Laakkonen, M.L. (2013) 'Efficacy of physical exercise intervention on mobility and physical functioning in older people with dementia: A systematic review.' *Experimental Gerontology 48*(1), 85–93.

Potter, R., Ellard, D., Rees, K. and Thorogood, M. (2011) 'A systematic review of the effects of physical activity on physical functioning, quality of life and depression in older people with dementia.' *International Journal of Geriatric Psychiatry 26*(10), 1000–1011.

Pringle, D. (2003) 'Making moments matter.' *Canadian Journal of Nursing Research* *35*(4), 7–13.

Rowe, J.W. and Kahn, R.L. (1997) 'Successful ageing.' *The Gerontologist 37*(4), 433–440.

Ryff, C.D. (1989a) 'Happiness is everything, or is it? Explorations on the meaning of psychological well-being.' *Journal of Personality and Social Psychology 57*(6), 1069–1081.

Ryff, C.D. (1989b) 'In the eye of the beholder: Views of psychological well-being among middle-aged and older adults.' *Psychology and Ageing 4*(2), 195–210.

Schulz, R., Cook, T.B., Beach, S.R., Lingler, J.H. *et al.* (2013) 'Magnitude and causes of bias among family caregivers rating Alzheimer disease patients.' *The American Journal of Geriatric Psychiatry 21*(1), 14–25.

Sixsmith, A. and Gibson, G. (2007) 'Music and the wellbeing of people with dementia.' *Ageing and Society 27*(1), 127–145.

Steeman, E., Casterlé, D., Dierckx, B., Godderis, J. and Grypdonck, M. (2006) 'Living with early-stage dementia: A review of qualitative studies.' *Journal of Advanced Nursing 54*(6), 722–738.

Steeman, E., Godderis, J., Grypdonck, M., De Bal, N. and De Casterlé, B.D. (2007) 'Living with dementia from the perspective of older people: Is it a positive story?' *Ageing and Mental Health 11*(2), 119–130.

Strawbridge, W.J., Wallhagen, M.I. and Cohen, R.D. (2002) 'Successful ageing and well-being self-rated compared with Rowe and Kahn.' *The Gerontologist 42*(6), 727–733.

Trigg, R., Skevington, S.M. and Jones, R.W. (2007) 'How can we best assess the quality of life of people with dementia? The Bath Assessment of Subjective Quality of Life in Dementia (BASQID).' *The Gerontologist 47*(6), 789–797.

van der Roest, H.G., Meiland, F.J., Maroccini, R., Comijs, H.C., Jonker, C. and Dröes, R.M. (2007) 'Subjective needs of people with dementia: A review of the literature.' *International Psychogeriatrics 19*(3), 559–592.

Venturato, L. (2010) 'Dignity, dining and dialogue: Reviewing the literature on quality of life for people with dementia.' *International Journal of Older People Nursing 5*(3), 228–234.

von Kutzleben, M., Schmid, W., Halek, M., Holle, B. and Bartholomeyczik, S. (2012) 'Community-dwelling persons with dementia: What do they need? What do they demand? What do they do? A systematic review on the subjective experiences of persons with dementia.' *Ageing and Mental Health 16*(3), 378–390.

Wiersma, E.C. and Pedlar, A. (2008) 'The nature of relationships in alternative dementia care environments.' *Canadian Journal on Ageing/La Revue Canadienne du Vieillissement 27*(1), 101–108.

Windle, G., Hughes, D., Linck, P., Russell, I. and Woods, B. (2010) 'Is exercise effective in promoting mental well-being in older age? A systematic review.' *Ageing and Mental Health 14*(6), 652–669.

Zeilig, H., Killick, J. and Fox, C. (2014) 'The participative arts for people living with a dementia: A critical review.' *International Journal of Ageing and Later Life 9*(1), 7–34.

Chapter 4

HOPE AND DEMENTIA

Emma Wolverson and Chris Clarke

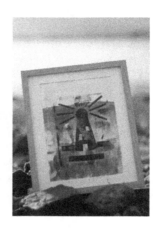

Hope is a construct that, at first glance, readers may well feel familiar with. The word 'hope' is commonly used in our everyday conversations, both as a noun and a verb. Hope permeates the worlds of philosophy, poetry and theology. It even extends to mythology – some readers will know of the myth of Pandora's Box, in which hope was the only spirit to remain in the box and make a difference when all the illnesses and hardships had escaped into the world. Hope is characterised as a precious and fragile asset but also, paradoxically, as a source of great strength and transformative power.

Whilst it has a 'common sense' quality, hope can also be elusive and difficult to define in scientific terms. In its simplest form, hope has been described as believing in the possibility of 'a positive future compared to a difficult present' (Duggleby *et al.*, 2010, p.150), but this definition may not capture its full emotional, existential and spiritual qualities. Hope has been regarded as an innate and fundamental feature of human life, without which life would not be possible (Frankl, 1963). Yet, at the same time, few other constructs are as divisive. Whilst the majority of people attest to hope being inherently beneficial, a vocal minority of dissenters have questioned its conceptual and adaptive value. Some are merely sceptical, suggesting that hope is perhaps too soft or vague a concept to be clinically useful. Others have questioned the conceit that hope is intrinsic or achievable and see 'genuine hope as rare and great', whilst warning instead of 'positive illusions' and 'false hope' (Tillich, 1965, p.17). More extreme voices have discredited hope as maladaptive, warning of its potential role as a bar to accepting unwanted eventualities (Tomko, 1985). In this way, hope is seen as that something that 'prolongs whatever torments us' (Nietzsche, 1986, p.45).

With these debates and controversies in mind, this chapter will examine how hope has been conceptualised within healthcare, before going on to consider the role of hope in later life and in living with an illness. Using this as a frame of reference, the chapter will then explore the construct in relation to dementia, focusing particularly on whether it is possible and important for people living with dementia to experience hope.

DEFINING HOPE IN HEALTHCARE

Where there's life, there's hope.

Marcus Tullius Cicero

It is often said that wherever there is life, there is hope. Perhaps echoing this proverb, hope has had a long tradition in the healthcare arena, but the scientific study of hope only really took off in the latter part of the 20th century. In relation to health, hope has come to be conceptualised as a complex, dynamic and multi-dimensional concept that continues to change over the life-span and across important life events, such as illness and ageing (Duggleby *et al.*, 2012). There has been multi-disciplinary interest in hope over the years, resulting in as many as 49 different empirical definitions and 32 standardised measures of hope (Schrank, Stanghellini and Slade, 2008). It has variously been regarded as: 'a cognitive set, based on a reciprocally derived sense of successful agency, that is, goal-directed determination and pathways (such as planning) to meet goals' (Snyder *et al.*, 1991, p.570); an emotion (Averill, Catlin and Chon, 1990); 'a relational process' (Marcel, 1962); and a trait-like personal strength reflecting an ability to find new meanings in life (Peterson and Seligman, 2004). Some have suggested that hope is particularly linked with a person's sense of meaning in life and that there may be a religious or spiritual structure underpinning hope (Dufault and Martochhio, 1985; Farran and McCann, 1989; Frankl, 1963).

ATTRIBUTES OF HOPE

Divergences in conceptualisations of hope highlight its multi-dimensional nature. At the same time, commonalties between definitions are evident and point towards what might be its central elements:

- *A context of uncertainty:* Hope may be a personal trait but is commonly seen as a response to trial or suffering that is present during times of crisis, loss, hardship, decision making and future planning.

- *Future orientation:* Hope is frequently described as a positive future orientation, that is, looking forward to a future that is good.

- *Goal focus:* Objects of hope may be specific and related to defined – 'hoped for' – goals; or it may relate to more generalised hopes, such as that life will be worth living in the future; or it may relate to spiritual/worldly domains. These objects of hope are accompanied by a sense of desire or longing – that which is hoped for is valued by and important to the person.

- *Based in reality:* A feature of hope that readily distinguishes it from its peers, optimism and wishing, is that the objects of hope are based in reality – that which is hoped for is in some sense realistic. However, definitions are not clear in stipulating whose reality hopes must be based in – that of the hoping person themselves or of those holding more powerful positions around them.

- *Energy:* For the hopeful person, hope is commonly seen as both requiring and providing a sense of force or energy that motivates a person to move away from their current context towards a positive future. In this way, a person is seen as active in the hoping process, yet also empowered by it. Hope is seen to strengthen, renew and invigorate people, and can increase feelings of confidence and control over uncertainty.

- *Involving others:* The value of others in the hoping process is commonly highlighted. The focus of hope often involves others, and hope is also commonly regarded as occurring between people, with the views and reactions of others often being cited as frequent barriers and facilitators to hope.

. . . .

Across its varying conceptualisations, hope is consistently cited as having the potential to influence both the quality and quantity of a person's life, and has been regarded as a prerequisite to effective coping and adaptation (Herth, 1993). It is thought to predict subjective well-being even after controlling for variance due to self-efficacy and optimism (Magaletta and Oliver, 1999); and higher hope has been consistently related to better physical health (see Snyder, Rand and Sigmon, 2005), adjustment (see Linley and Joseph, 2004) and effective psychotherapy (see Bergin and Walsh, 2005). As such, hope is now ingrained within the concept of caring (Stephenson, 1991), with growing recognition of its therapeutic value in recovery (Hobbs and Baker, 2012).

HOPE IN LATER LIFE

McFadden, Ingram and Baldauf (2001) state that holding onto hope about ageing is an enormous challenge for both individuals and societies. They highlight how most Western cultures are 'split' between unrealistic hope and morbid pessimism about ageing. Much of the literature on hope and ageing is, unfortunately, consistent with the latter position, which inadvertently underpins and maintains ageism. Later life is often regarded as a time that brings a number of challenges to maintaining hope, such as the accumulation of losses and health problems that contribute to a decreasing ability to care for oneself. As such, the ageing process itself is seen to block pathways, render goals unattainable and cause a person to lose motivation and agency to pursue 'hoped for' goals (Cheavens and Gum, 2000). In interviews with 60 older people, Herth (1993) identified a number of barriers to hope in later life including depleted energy, uncontrollable pain and suffering in oneself or the world as well as, notably, impaired cognition. Simply being closer to death might also be seen to negate hope, given its focus on the future. Indeed, as a construct, hope is typically orientated towards younger adults, whose futures are regarded as more open-ended. Older people, and perhaps particularly those living with dementia, are often viewed as more preoccupied with the past than they are focused on achieving goals in the future.

If we subscribe to this view that ageing represents a threat to hope, then the task for the individual in the face of negative and challenging losses is to seek to maintain hope. This could perhaps take the form of trying to adapt to or compensate for blocked pathways to goals, problem-solve to find new ways to reach 'hoped for' goals, or perhaps form new hopes. Some models of successful ageing indicate the possible mechanisms by which this could occur and, in doing so, help challenge the notion that ageing and hope are mutually exclusive. Such models increasingly recognise the subjective nature of successful ageing; only older people themselves can rate the extent to which they are ageing successfully (cf. Cernin, Lysack and Lichtenberg, 2011). Cheavens and Gum (2000) contend that hope plays a powerful role in ageing successfully and that successful ageing is also associated with continued levels of high hope in the later stages of life. In support, Araújo and colleagues (2015) found that those older people who considered themselves to be ageing successfully tended to be higher in self-efficacy, purpose in life and hope. Like successful ageing, then, hope in later life is subjective and does not appear dependent on health status or functional ability (Herth, 1993).

Whilst some have argued that the notion of successful ageing can engender false hopes by implying a degree of personal control that may not be realistic in later life (Katz and Marshall, 2004), it can be argued that the mere presence of discourses around ageing successfully offers new hopes to older people by bestowing upon them a sense of agency and purpose and by challenging the prevailing view of later life as a hopeless time. Furthermore, models of successful ageing remind us that ageing is not something that happens overnight but is in fact a life-long process (Pruchno, Heid and Genderson, 2015). Older people have overcome challenges and engaged in growth and adaptation across their entire life-spans. Why then would someone who has been hoping for positive futures their whole life, suddenly stop hoping for a meaningful end to it? The end of life for many is not an event but often a process, which is now set in a context of heightened uncertainty. Given this, hope is an even more important resource for the person to draw on to help deal with the challenges of life (Cutcliffe and Herth, 2002; Duggleby *et al.*, 2012).

Erikson (1977; also see Erikson, Erikson and Kivnivk, 1986) places hope firmly within this developmental context, positing that hope is learned in infancy but evolves throughout the life cycle. Supporting this notion, Westburg (1999) reported that attachment experiences in early life predicted levels of maintained hope in a sample of 17 older women. However, Erikson did not see levels of hope as set in childhood. His theory of psycho-social development implies that hope can increase at any age and that the adversities a person might experience in later life could actually serve as stimuli for hope. He noted that older people gain hope by balancing feelings of despair with a sense of ego integrity, as they engage in a search for meaning and purpose through a process of life review. He further proposed that if a person is able to achieve integrity and reflect on their life as having been rich and meaningful, their hope may then extend beyond themselves and their current circumstances and become directed towards others, thus reflecting the development of generativity. Supporting this notion, research has suggested that older people not only hope for personal good health and autonomy but also a continued sense of connectedness to others (Lapierre, Bouffard and Bastin, 1997; Rapkin and Fisher, 1992). As such, older people may have multiple and co-existing hopes that relate to others or the world rather than themselves. Moreover, hopes in later life may relate to a more immediate future (weeks, days), a future that it less well-defined or even a future extending beyond this life (Duggleby *et al.*, 2010).

These issues indicate that individualistic notions of hope grounded in achievement and success may be problematic and limiting for older people (Farran, Salloway and Clark, 1990). Accordingly, in defining hope in later life, Dufault and Martocchio (1985) emphasise its multi-dimensional and process-orientated nature by proposing two spheres of hope: 'particularised hope' relates to a defined object or goals, whilst 'generalised hope' implies a sense of a positive future that extends beyond the limitations of time and serves to protect against despair when a person may be deprived of particular hopes, whether by themselves, their situation or by those around them. Generalised hope therefore preserves or restores a sense of meaning and motivation in later life when particular forms of hope are blocked. Similarly, Herth (1993, p.151) defined hope in later life as 'an inner power that facilitates transcendence of the present situation and enables a reality-based expectation of a brighter tomorrow for self and/or others'.

Growing evidence attests to the active presence of hope in the experiences of older people, regardless of age, gender, health and functional ability (cf. Chimich and Nekolaichuk, 2004; Davis, 2005). Research has also highlighted how older people employ different methods of maintaining hope when compared with younger people and that, in later life, maintaining hope is an active process that arises from both within and outside a person. Faced with the reality of a 'downward trajectory' (Farran, Salloway and Clarke, 1990), older adults use particular cognitive–behavioural strategies to maintain hope, such as drawing inner strength from positive memories or positive affirmations (Herth, 1993). Crucially though, maintaining hope also involves reaching out to others to make meaningful connections with people and engaging in activities that are meaningful and which provide both a sense of purpose and a wider connection with the universe (Duggleby *et al.*, 2012; Herth, 1993). Hope in later life, then, is maintained through a multitude of means, all of which have clear implications for interventions and environments designed to foster hope.

HOPE IN ILLNESS

In healthcare, clinicians measure and monitor levels of hope in relation to people's experiences of illness and take action to support, sustain and enhance it if it is threatened or waning. Clinicians may even act as temporary guardians of hope for those who are vulnerable, particularly in circumstances where hope is deemed to be lost or unattainable. This responsibility almost becomes a moral imperative when one recognises the value of hope in chronic illness, which is now well established. Hope has been regarded as essential in regaining and maintaining health and promoting wellness (Herth, 1992) and is associated with better adjustment and coping in a range of health conditions (e.g. Snyder, Rand and Sigmon, 2005). People who are more hopeful demonstrate more compliance with recommended treatments (Good *et al.*, 1990), use more information about their illness (Snyder *et al.*, 2000), experience less pain (Snyder, Odle and Hackman, 1999) and report more benefit finding in their illness experience (Affleck and Tennen, 1996).

However, what is less clear in this literature is how hope contributes to these outcomes and what it is that people living with a chronic health condition may best hope for when they may be contending with a series of threats to hope including uncontrollable pain, a devaluation of personhood, disablement and untimely death (Wilkinson, 1996). Under these circumstances, hoping for a cure would be natural, but is at the same time problematic. Some writers have suggested that hope exists along a continuum, with hope for a cure at the outset being reframed as a person moves to the end of life (Pattison and Lee, 2009). At this stage, people may engage in hoping that is directed more towards finding meaning from and transcending their illness. These possibilities highlight two distinct discourses surrounding hope in relation to illness: one concerning hope for a cure and another concerning meaning in life (Duggleby *et al.*, 2010), each of which will now be explored in turn.

HOPE FOR A CURE

The discourse of hope for a cure is particularly striking within the context of cancer care. For many years, 'The Big C' was considered a taboo topic in much the same way people might struggle to talk openly about dementia today. Good and colleagues (1990) suggest that a discourse of hope for a cure now underpins the entire enterprise of cancer research and treatment. The belief that cancer can be cured, if not now then in the future, is central to research-funding and providing hope to those living with cancer, and the idea that we will ultimately *defeat* cancer has radically changed the way we talk about it. The use of war as a dominant enabling metaphor has arguably created hope where there once was none. Framing cancer as an external aggressor that attacks and invades people's bodies separates the person from the illness and positions people living with it as responsible for their own hope in fighting their illness (Elliot and Oliver, 2009). Hope is created and maintained by a person's determination to courageously keep fighting and, of course, not lose.

There are clear limitations to such an implicitly power-based and violent discourse (Mitchell, Ferguson-Pare and Richards, 2003). Research consistently suggests that conflict, fighting and war are not usually people's preferred ways of coping with illness (Hawkins, 1999), perhaps because these effectively amount to declaring war on oneself. Others would argue that the rhetoric of hope as absolute victory through cure overshadows other valuable approaches to illness, such as rehabilitation and recovery (George and Whitehouse, 2014). Duggleby and colleagues (2010) argue that such messages are also ageist as they are invariably focused on curing young individuals, with the implicit assumption being that they have more to live for and hope for.

EXTENDING HOPE BEYOND A CURE

Even when they are aware of the reality of their situation, many people with a terminal illness hold onto the notion of hope for a cure or for a longer life (cf. Pattison and Lee, 2011). Yet there can be another level to hoping in these circumstances. Exploratory and descriptive studies examining the meaning and importance of hope for people at the end of their life have demonstrated how the focus and meaning of hope can extend far beyond narrow conceptualisations of hope for a cure. Rather than finding that people facing a terminal prognosis are without hope, the literature consistently supports the notion that hope is an important psychological resource as people die (Herth, 1990; Kubler-Ross, 1969). Herth (1990) found the degree of hope reported by cancer patients actually increased as signs of disease progression became more evident.

Hope has been observed to facilitate transcendence by allowing a person to look beyond their current difficulties to develop a new, broader awareness of others and the environment (Herth, 1990). Duggleby and colleagues (2012) suggest that in order to transcend a situation a person must look both inwards and to others in order to find meaning and purpose in life. Supporting this notion, Elliott and Oliver (2009) examined the socio-linguistic properties of hope in the speech of dying patients. They concluded that hope becomes a resource for those who are dying, not because people seek to defy death but because hope allows people to affirm life. Correspondingly, some have theorised that the main function of hope is to serve as an emergency virtue (Lynch 1965) to make life bearable in situations where needs and goals cannot be met.

The notion that hope in illness can represent a process of transcendence underpins the principles of the hospice movement, which has been important in recognising that hope for a cure is not the only legitimate hope. The hospice model of care emphasises that acceptance of a terminal illness is not seen as extinguishing hope but is, in fact, essential to achieving it.

In order to maintain hope in illness, people are thought to go through a process of re-appraisal that enables them to let go of old hopes whilst also seeing positive possibilities in their future (Dufault and Martocchio, 1985; Duggleby and Wright, 2005; Elliot and Oliver, 2009). This may result in finding new hopes, such as hope for peace and comfort, rather than hope for a cure. The timely sharing of prognostic information is important to this process as it can facilitate the formation of 'realistic hopes'. Hinds and Martin (1988) describe how, when living with a terminal illness, hope will alter as the person accepts and adapts to their diagnosis. During this time, denial, light-heartedness and humour may play an important role in allowing a person the necessary time to adapt and refocus their hopes. This process also takes place in an interpersonal and social context; re-evaluating hopes is facilitated by reaching out and connecting with families, friends, healthcare professionals and spiritual figures, allowing people to take a broader perspective of what is happening (Duggleby *et al.*, 2012; Herth, 1990; Elliot and Oliver, 2009). The need to be connected to others is significant because it highlights how hope in these situations can be carried collectively. Weingarten (2000) stated that hope is ultimately the responsibility of a community. This clearly has implications for illnesses that carry significant social stigma such as HIV/AIDS and, of course, dementia.

DEMENTIA – DARING TO HOPE

The concept of hope in dementia has, so far, received very little attention within healthcare research (Cotter, 2009). The idea of applying hope to the experience of dementia is possibly counter-intuitive for many, at clinical and societal levels. The prevailing view of dementia in society tends strongly towards hopelessness as dominant discourses and media images have consistently framed dementia as a tragedy in which a person is lost in the worst possible way (see Behuniak, 2011; Peel, 2014). Dementia therefore typically engenders a deep and pernicious fear in our society and, echoing discourses on cancer, is often framed as an external menace to be defeated, with the ultimate hope for a technical cure continually reinforced both by media coverage and international health policy initiatives, such as the G8 Dementia Summit Declaration, 2013 (Department of Health, 2013).

In the absence of this cure, cholinesterase inhibitors have been afforded almost mythical status by the media, and a crucial task for clinicians working in memory and healthcare services has therefore been to manage expectations when prescribing them. There has been growing recognition of the need for sensitivity and careful negotiation when withdrawing these drugs where they are not effective, or have become ineffective, to ensure that this is not seen as abandoning hope (Prakash and Thacker, 2014). In the absence of a cure and in the face of social stigma, attending a memory clinic and seeking a diagnosis is, in itself, an act of hope for some. It has been argued that the memory clinic movement risks creating false hope for people who have dementia, because of the drive towards early detection and diagnosis in the absence of a cure and, crucially, adequate support services (Coombes, 2009). However, there is growing recognition that the provision of accurate and timely information facilitates a grounding in reality that is essential for hope by challenging stigma and misinformation (Moniz-Cook and Manthorpe, 2008).

People living with dementia face further barriers to experiencing and maintaining hope that emanate from dementia itself. For example, Snyder's (2002) cognitive theory of hope suggests that hope is, primarily, a way of thinking, thus implying that it requires a number of intellectual skills such as abstract reasoning, planning, cognitive flexibility and attention, which may be problematic, if not unachievable, for a person living with dementia. Several theories of hope also recognise the role of memory (Dufault and Martocchio, 1985; Groopman, 2004); hopefulness can involve integrating information from present circumstances and past experiences with the experiences of other individuals who endured and overcame difficult situations. If hope is seen as a learned process (Erikson, 1977), then perhaps in dementia it becomes vulnerable to unlearning and loss, along with other skills. Furthermore, cognitive changes may threaten a person's ability to re-evaluate hopes based on a realistic appraisal of one's circumstances.

Key challenges for people who have dementia therefore relate to whether hope can be retained when cognitive skills and awareness have changed, and whether it may continue to exist at a subjective or behavioural level in spite of dementia. Significantly, Kitwood and Bredin (1992) argued that this is possible and that hope functions as one of four global states that underpin subjective and relative well-being in dementia, each dependent on the quality of the social environment.

The positive psychology construct of Character Strengths and Virtues (see Peterson and Seligman, 2004) complements this in framing hope as a trait-like personal strength connected with the personal virtue of transcendence. These perspectives imply that experiencing hopefulness could extend beyond changes in cognitive ability, potentially involving more generalised than particularised hopes.

Further challenges and potential losses in dementia may constitute barriers to retaining hope. Unlike other chronic illnesses, such as cancer (which is regarded as something that 'invades' a healthy body), dementia is seen as something that 'invades' a *person*. People living with dementia have not been seen as taking an active role in fighting their illness or as possessing the same sense of agency because of the historical view that the person as was is no longer there. People living with dementia have described a tension between holding onto their own identity and constructing a new one (Pearce, Clare and Pistrang, 2002). As discussed, hope in later life involves a sense of consolidation and holding onto an identity accrued over time. The challenge for people with dementia, therefore, might be seen in terms of retaining enough of a sense of agency and identity in order to make hopefulness possible.

Social environments are likely to be pivotal to this challenge. Sadly, we know that people with dementia can become vulnerable to malignant social environments that perpetrate stigmatisation and labelling, exclusion and disempowerment, which can undermine a sense of agency, identity and well-being. Hope also exists in a social context. Elliott (2005) argues that hope cannot be created or maintained by individuals in isolation but requires ongoing positive social interactions to endure, a notion highly relevant to dementia care. Cutcliffe and Grant (2001) suggest that dementia-care nurses can inspire and instil hope through humanistic care practices. In support, Spector and Orrell (2006) reported a significant link between hope in residential care staff and higher quality of life in people living with dementia. Whilst living with dementia poses a number of challenges to hope, perhaps the biggest lies not in the absence of a cure or even a person's cognitive capacity, but in the degree to which a person's social environment can support and sustain hopefulness. To date there has only been one study exploring hope in relation to family caregivers of people living with dementia. Duggleby and colleagues (2009) conducted a grounded theory study to explore the experience of hope for 17 family members caring for people with dementia. Dementia was framed as a threat to hope, and caregivers shared fears of losing hope. In order to maintain their hope, family caregivers went through a continual process of renewing it each day. The authors interpreted this process in terms of three related themes: coming to terms (acknowledging the reality of the situation), finding positives (including connecting with others) and seeing different possibilities.

HOW CAN PEOPLE WITH DEMENTIA BUILD HOPE?

The challenges to hope in dementia that we have outlined are profound. Yet, in general, research on hope consistently concludes that some degree of hope is present in nearly all people and only rarely do people report that they are completely hopeless, even when living with chronic and terminal illnesses (Nowotny, 1989). So how might we come to understand hope in the experience of dementia?

Literature on the lived experience of dementia, often based on phenomenological and constructionist perspectives, is highly pertinent to answering this question. People with dementia and their caregivers have described a range of ways they cope in their everyday lives and re-assign meaning to their experiences. Throughout this literature there exist accounts of people expecting the best and maintaining a positive outlook on life and the future (Gillies, 2000; MacRae, 2010; Mok *et al.*, 2007), consistent with the future orientation aspect of hope that is central to most theories (see earlier in the chapter). A sense of determination and agency to live life to the full in spite of a diagnosis of dementia is also echoed within this literature (Clare, 2002; Gillies, 2000; Harman and Clare, 2006; Nygard and Borell, 1998). Framing people with dementia as active in facing and fighting their illness suggests that they may also be active in the process of hoping rather than passively waiting for a cure, or succumbing to despair. Accepting dementia as a part of one's life appears to be key in learning to live with it and, in turn, maintaining hope has been described as key to acceptance as it can allow people to focus on upholding meaning and purpose in their lives rather than dwelling exclusively on their illness (Werezak and Stewart 2002).

Our own work in this emerging area is concerned with exploring the meaning and experience of hope in older people living with dementia as well as the barriers and facilitators to hopefulness in this context

(Wolverson, Clarke and Moniz-Cook, 2010). Since previous lived experience studies that have found evidence of experiences relating to hopefulness have done so serendipitously, we carried out an exploratory phenomenological study to directly investigate the lived experience of hope in ten older people with the early stages of dementia. The themes that emerged reflected shared as well as contrasting meanings of hope among participants.

What follows is a summary of the main findings of this study, including representative quotes from people living with dementia who took part (for more detailed results, see Wolverson, Clarke and Moniz-Cook, 2010).

. . . .   **OVERARCHING THEMES**

1. LIVE IN HOPE OR DIE IN DESPAIR

This theme reflected how participants managed a tension between hope-fostering beliefs, built over the life-span, and hope-hindering life experiences in living with dementia. This involved a balancing process where the re-appraisal of hopes, based on the reality of hope-hindering experiences associated with both old age and dementia, led to renewed hopefulness and contentment:

> You always hope for something better, but I don't see how it can get better. I am quite content as I am now.
>
> *(Participant 3)*

Above all, hope appeared to be a vital presence in the lives of the participants. In contrast to the various challenges to hope posed by a dementia diagnosis (as outlined above), our study participants did not talk much about hope having been changed or challenged, and many denied ever losing hope at all. Instead, hope was described as something intrinsic and innate that could not be lost because it was a fundamental part of being human, as illustrated simply by this quote:

> Well, I think it's natural to have hope.
>
> *(Participant 8)*

Participants situated hope firmly within a life-span perspective, linking it clearly with their own attachment histories, spiritual beliefs and experiences. Participants used reminiscence to draw on autobiographical memories of survival and success, which allowed them to recapture previous strengths and create an attitude of resilience:

> I think I have seen life you know.
>
> *(Participant 5)*

> I don't really know...I think it was my father, I think he hoped for everything. I feel as if I'm a lot like him. He was a skipper on the trawlers; he always knew what he wanted and what he wanted to do and I think that's a little bit of me. If I want to do it, I will do it; and if I don't want to do [it], I won't.
>
> *(Participant 6)*

Consistent with definitions of generalised versus particularised hope within the literature (Dufault and Martocchio, 1985) participants did not talk about attaining specific hopes. In fact, people described hoping *for* less:

> I mean a lot of older folk don't want the same.
>
> *(Participant 7)*

For these participants then, hope was described as a belief that there is always something better, and it provided a way of helping people to live in the present. There were very few reports of future-orientated hope, and where this existed it mostly related to passing on a legacy of hope for a better future for family and society:

> I mean my hopes now are for my son and his wife and their two boys.
>
> *(Participant 10)*

Only one participant described hope for a cure, although they stated that this was a false hope:

> They haven't come up with a cure for memory yet and I don't think they will.
>
> *(Participant 1)*

Instead, hope was described as an approach to life that engenders a sense of energy and that mobilises people in the present. This hopeful attitude allowed people to frame both dementia and ageing as challenges and allowed participants to consider the future by looking at ways to take steps in the present to move beyond their current situation towards something better:

> I can't really see this condition getting any better. But I
> have started: it's a little step, but I have started going to
> the gym.
>
> *(Participant 8)*

Overlapping with studies exploring barriers to hope in later life, participants spoke about a number of challenges to their hope that they faced in daily life, such as increasing dependency, awareness of making mistakes, a loss of confidence and changes in social relationships including loss of role, respect, isolation and loneliness:

> I tend to get left out a bit – not because anybody intended
> to do that, they just don't hear.
>
> *(Participant 8)*

At the same time, participants spoke of balancing their inherent tendency to hope for something better with a degree of acceptance about their current situation. Many stated that they had made peace with their circumstances:

> On the whole I haven't done so bad for myself.
>
> *(Participant 9)*

2. KEEP LIVING AND KEEP LIVING WELL

This overarching theme describes the positive attitudes towards health and social circumstances that emerged from successfully balancing the tension between hope-fostering beliefs and hope-hindering experiences in living with dementia. Through this process, hope was maintained actively through key coping behaviours and was focused on keeping healthy and maintaining relationships with others and the world.

Key to maintaining a good quality of life for all participants was the hope to keep healthy. This related to both their physical health and a hope that their memory would remain intact for as long as possible. Participants described good health as vital to all their other hopes:

> I mean, without good health there is nothing.
>
> *(Participant 4)*

Keeping healthy was regarded as vital to remaining independent and being able to continue to carry out activities of daily living. Independence elicited a strong sense of hope in participants, and remaining independent in activities of daily living was a hope expressed by all participants:

...that I can do my own housework, pay my own bills. That's just what I hope for until I die.

(Participant 6)

All participants expressed a hope to stay connected to other people, particularly their family. The importance of family, and in particular maintaining regular contact with their children, was notable in maintaining hope:

Without her [daughter], I don't think I'd be here now.

(Participant 5)

Social contact was often cited as important for maintaining hope. In fact, two participants asked the interviewer if more chances to meet people could be arranged:

I just wondered if another afternoon out might make me brighter.

(Participant 7)

Hope was described as an ingredient necessary for enhancing the quality of each day through engendering positive attitudes to coping. One such attitude described by many participants was the importance of taking one day at a time:

You live for the day.

(Participant 9)

All participants also spoke about the importance of 'keeping busy' and how this helped to maintain their hope. Participants spoke about using activity when they felt low in hope:

You know, if I'm feeling low, I think: 'Is there anything I could be doing?'

(Participant 2)

The most important way to keep busy was described as getting out of the house and taking part in a pleasurable activity:

I'm going out more nowadays. Going out more is the best thing to do.

(Participant 7)

. . . .

The study's findings strongly suggest that hope is a relevant and important concept for people living with dementia despite the real challenges they face (e.g. cognitive impairment, exclusion, disempowerment). Hope was experienced mostly in generalised terms and often directed towards the well-being of others, suggesting the relevance of a life-span developmental perspective. Hopes for others and for continued health and quality of life overshadowed hopes for a cure for dementia. In addition, hope was identified as an innate approach to living in the here-and-now that allowed the participants to keep going, echoing its conceptualisation as a trait-like personal strength but indicating that the degree of future orientation in hopefulness in dementia does change. Overall, participants appeared to be active in maintaining their hope by negotiating the tension between hope-fostering attitudes and hope-hindering experiences.

CONCLUSIONS

As Snyder (2001) so eloquently said, 'the perseverance of hope can indeed form the bridge that links our common humanity to persons with Alzheimer's' (p.19). And so, while much has yet to be learnt about the role of hope and its impact on dementia, it seems evident that investigating hope and honouring its presence in people's experiences of dementia is an important aspect of a person-centred approach to research and care that highlights our shared humanity.

Perhaps we are able to say at this point that we have re-opened Pandora's Box in order to gain a deeper understanding of hope and its potential relevance to dementia. Hope is a motivating and protective personal strength that develops across the life-span, becoming less goal-focused and future-focused in later life and in dementia, yet no less vital. Hope can extend beyond a cure, and in dementia it is connected with preserving meaning, social connectedness and a sense of purpose. In this chapter we suggest that we have not released further 'evils' into the world of dementia care by exploring hope but have instead demonstrated the relevance of this complex concept to understanding how a person might live well with dementia.

REFERENCES

Affleck, G. and Tennen, H. (1996) 'Constructing benefits from adversity: Adaptational significance and dispositional underpinnings.' *Journal of Personality 64*, 899–922.

Araújo, L., Ribeiro, O., Teixeira, L. and Paúl, C. (2015) 'Successful aging at 100 years: The relevance of subjectivity and psychological resources.' *International Psychogeriatrics 28*(2), 179–188.

Averill, J.R., Catlin, G. and Chon, K.K. (1990) *Rules of Hope*. New York, NY: Springer.

Behuniak, S.M. (2011) 'The living dead? The construction of people with Alzheimer's disease as zombies.' *Ageing and Society 31*(1), 70–92.

Bergin, L. and Walsh, S. (2005) 'The role of hope in psychotherapy with older adults.' *Aging and Mental Health 9*(1), 7–15.

Cernin, P., Lysack, C. and Lichtenberg, P. (2011) 'A comparison of self-rated and objectively measured successful aging constructs in an urban sample of African American older adults.' *Clinical Gerontologist 34*, 89–102.

Cheavens, J. and Gum, A. (2000) 'Gray Power: Hope for the Ages.' In C. Snyder (ed.) *Handbook of Hope: Theory, Measures, and Applications*. San Diego, CA: Academic Press.

Chimich, W. and Nekolaichuk, C. (2004) 'Exploring the links between depression, integrity, and hope in the elderly.' *Canadian Journal of Psychiatry 49*(7), 428–433.

Clare, L. (2002) 'We'll fight it as long as we can: Coping with the onset of Alzheimer's disease.' *Aging and Mental Health 6*, 139–148.

Coombes, R. (2009) 'Evidence lacking for memory clinics to tackle dementia, say critics.' *British Medical Journal 338*, b550.

Cotter, V. (2009) 'Hope in early-stage dementia: A concept analysis.' *Alzheimer's Care Today 14*(4), 232–237.

Cutcliffe, J.R. and Grant, G. (2001) 'What are the principles and processes of inspiring hope in cognitively impaired older adults within a continuing care environment?' *Journal of Psychiatric and Mental Health Nursing 8*, 427–436.

Cutcliffe, J. and Herth, K. (2002) 'The concept of hope in nursing 2: Hope and mental health nursing.' *British Journal of Nursing 11*(13), 885–893.

Davis, B. (2005) 'Mediators of the relationship between hope and well-being in older adults.' *Clinical Nursing Research 14*(3), 253–272.

Department of Health (2013) *G8 dementia summit declaration*. Available at www.gov.uk/government/publications/g8-dementia-summit-agreements, accessed on 15 April 2016.

Dufault, K. and Martocchio, B. (1985) 'Hope: Its spheres and dimensions.' *Nursing Clinics of North America 20*(2), 379–391.

Duggleby, W., Hicks, D., Nekolaichuk, C., Holtslander, L. *et al.* (2012) 'Hope, older adults, and chronic illness: A metasynthesis of qualitative research.' *Journal of Advanced Nursing 68*(6), 1211–1223.

Duggleby, W., Holtslander, L., Kylma, J., Duncan, V., Hammond, C. and Williams, A. (2010) 'Metasynthesis of the hope experience of family caregivers of persons with chronic illness.' *Qualitative Health Research 20*(2), 148–158.

Duggleby, W. and Wright, K. (2005) 'Transforming hope: How elderly palliative patients live with hope.' *Canadian Journal of Nursing Research 37*(2), 70–84.

Duggleby, W., Williams, A., Wright, K. and Bollinger, S. (2009) 'Renewing everyday hope: The hope experience of family caregivers of persons with dementia.' *Issues in Mental Health Nursing 30*(8), 514–521.

Eliott, J.A. (2005) *Interdisciplinary Perspectives on Hope*. Hauppauge, NY: Nova Science Publishers.

Eliott, J. and Oliver, I. (2009) 'Hope, life, and death: A qualitative analysis of dying cancer patients' talk about hope.' *Death Studies 33*, 609–638.

Erikson, E. (1977) *Childhood and Society*. London: Paladine.

Erikson, E., Erikson, J. and Kivnivk, H. (1986) *Vital Involvement in Old Age*. New York, NY: Norton.

Farran, C.J. and McCann, J. (1989) 'Longitudinal analysis of hope in community-based older adults.' *Archives in Psychiatric Nursing 3*, 272–276.

Farran, C., Salloway, J. and Clark, D. (1990) 'Measurement of hope in a community-based older population.' *Western Journal of Nursing Research 12*(1), 42–59.

Frankl, V.E. (1963) *Man's Search for Meaning. An Introduction to Logotherapy. From Death-camp to Existentialism*. Boston: Beacon Press.

George, D. and Whitehouse, P. (2004) 'The war (on terror) on Alzheimer's.' *Dementia 13*(1), 120–130.

Gillies, B.A. (2000) 'A memory like clockwork: Accounts of living through dementia.' *Aging and Mental Health 4*, 366–374.

Good, M., Good, B., Schaffer, C. and Lind, S. (1990) 'American oncology and the discourse of hope.' *Culture, Medicine and Society 14*(1), 59–79.

Groopman, J. (2004) *The Anatomy of Hope: How You Can Find Strength in the Face of Illness*. London: Simon & Schuster.

Harman, G. and Clare, L. (2006) 'Illness representations and lived experience in early stage dementia.' *Qualitative Health Research 16*, 484–502.

Hawkins, A. (1999) *Reconstructing Illness: Studies in Pathography* (2nd edn). West Lafayette, IN: Perdue University Press.

Herth, K. (1990) 'Fostering hope in terminally ill people.' *Journal of Advanced Nursing 15*, 1250–1259.

Herth, K. (1992) 'An abbreviated instrument to measure hope: Development and psychometric evaluation.' *Journal of Advanced Nursing 17*, 1251–1259.

Herth, K. (1993) 'Hope in older adults in community and institutional settings.' *Issues in Mental Health Nursing 14*(2), 139–156.

Hinds, P. and Martin, J. (1988) 'Hopefulness and the self-sustaining process in adolescents with cancer.' *Nursing Research 37*(6), 336–339.

Hobbs, M. and Baker, M. (2012) 'Hope for recovery – how clinicians may facilitate this in their work.' *Journal of Mental Health 21*(2), 144–153.

Katz, S. and Marshall, B. (2004) 'Is the functional "normal"? Aging, sexuality and the bio-marking of successful living.' *History of the Human Sciences 17*(1), 53–75.

Kitwood, T. and Bredin, K. (1992) 'Towards a theory of dementia care: Personhood and well-being.' *Ageing and Society 12*(3), 269–287.

Kubler-Ross, E. (1969) *On Death and Dying*. London: Tavistock.

Lapierre, S., Bouffard, L. and Bastin, E. (1997) 'Personal goals and subjective well-being in later life.' *International Journal of Geriatric Psychiatry 13*, 707–716.

Linley, P. and Joseph, S. (2004) 'Positive change following trauma and adversity: A review.' *Journal of Traumatic Stress 17*, 11–21.

Lynch, W.F. (1965) *Images of Hope: Imagination as Healer of the Hopeless*. Baltimore, MD: Helicon.

MacRae, H. (2010) 'Managing identity while living with Alzheimer's disease.' *Qualitative Health Research 20*(3), 293–305.

Magaletta, P. and Oliver, J. (1999) 'The hope construct, will, and ways: Their relations with self-efficacy, optimism and general well-being.' *Journal of Clinical Psychology 55*, 539–551.

Marcel, G. (1962) *Homo Viator: Introduction to a Metaphysics on Hope* (translated by E. Crawford). New York: Harper & Row.

McFadden, S.H., Ingram, M. and Baldauf, C. (2001) 'Actions, feelings, and values: Foundations of meaning and personhood in dementia.' *Journal of Religious Gerontology 11*(3–4), 67–86.

Mitchell. G., Ferguson-Pare, M. and Richards, J. (2003) 'Exploring an alternative metaphor for nursing: Relinquishing military images and language.' *Canadian Journal of Nursing Leadership 16*, 48–58.

Mok, E., Lai, C.K.Y., Wong, F.L.F. and Wan, P. (2007) 'Living with early-stage dementia: The perspective of older Chinese people.' *Journal of Advanced Nursing 59*, 591–600.

Moniz-Cook, E. and Manthorpe, J. (2008) *Early Psychosocial Interventions in Dementia: Evidence-based Practice*. London: Jessica Kingsley.

Nietzsche, F. (1986) *Human, All Too Human* Vol. 1 (original work published 1878). (R.J. Hollingdale, Trans.). Cambridge: Cambridge University Press.

Nygard, L. and Borell, L. (1998) 'A life-world altering meaning: Expressions of the illness experience of dementia in every-day life over 3 years.' *The Occupational Therapy Journal of Research 18*, 109–136.

Nowotny, M.L. (1989) 'Assessment of hope in patients with cancer: Development of an instrument.' *Oncology Nursing Forum 16*(1), 57–61.

Pattison, N. and Lee, C. (2011) 'Hope against hope in cancer at the end of life.' *Journal of Religious Health 50*, 731–742.

Pearce, A., Clare, L. and Pistrang, N. (2002) 'Managing sense of self: Coping in the early stages of Alzheimer's disease.' *Dementia 1*(2), 173–192.

Peel, E. (2014) '"The living death of Alzheimer's" versus "Take a walk to keep dementia at bay": Representations of dementia in print media and carer discourse.' *Sociology of Health & Illness 36*(6), 885–901.

Peterson, C. and Seligman, M. (2004) *Character Strengths and Virtues: A Handbook and Classification*. New York, NY: Oxford University Press.

Prakash, A. and Thacker, S. (2014) 'The audacity of hope: Tyranny and liberation in dementia care.' Available at www.gmjournal.co.uk/The_audacity_of_hope_tyranny_or_liberation_in_dementia_care_25769811827.aspx, accessed on 15 April 2016.

Pruchno, R., Heid, A.R. and Genderson, M.W. (2015) 'Resilience and successful aging: Aligning complementary constructs using a life course approach.' *Psychological Inquiry 26*(2), 200–207.

Rapkin, B. and Fisher, A. (1992) 'Framing the construct of life satisfaction in terms of older adults' personal goals.' *Psychology and Aging 7*, 138–149.

Schrank, B., Stanghellini, G. and Slade, M. (2008) 'Hope in psychiatry: A review of the literature.' *Acta Psychiatria Scandinavica 118*(6), 421–433.

Snyder, L. (2001) 'The lived experience of Alzheimer's – understanding the feelings and subjective accounts of persons with the disease.' *Alzheimer's Care Quarterly 2*(2), 8–22.

Snyder, C.R. (2002) 'Hope theory: Rainbows in the mind.' *Psychological Inquiry 13*(4), 249–275.

Snyder, C., Feldman, D., Taylor, J., Schroeder, L. and Adams, V. (2000) 'The roles of hopeful thinking in preventing problems and enhancing strengths.' *Applied and Preventative Psychology 15*, 262–295.

Snyder, C., Harris, C., Anderson, J., Holleran, S. *et al.* (1991) 'The will and the ways: Development and validation of an individual-differences measure of hope.' *Journal of Personality and Social Psychology 60*(4), 570–585.

Snyder, C., Odle, C. and Hackman, J. (1999) *Hope as related to perceived severity and tolerance of physical pain.* Paper presented in August 1999 at the American Psychological Association, Boston, MA, USA.

Snyder, C., Rand, K. and Sigmon, D. (2005) 'Hope Theory: A Member of the Positive Psychology Family.' In C. Snyder and S. Lopez (eds) *Handbook of Positive Psychology.* New York, NY: Oxford University Press.

Spector, M. and Orrell, M. (2006) 'Quality of life in dementia: A comparison of the perception of people with dementia and care staff in residential homes.' *Alzheimer Disease and Associated Disorders 20*(3), 160–165.

Stephenson, C. (1991) 'The concept of hope revisited for nursing.' *Journal of Advanced Nursing 16*, 1456–1461.

Tillich, P. (1965) 'The right to hope.' *The University of Chicago Magazine 58*, 16–22.

Tomko, B. (1985) 'The burden of hope.' *Hospice Journal 1*(3), 91–97.

Weingarten, K. (2000) 'Witnessing, wonder, and hope.' *Family Process 39*, 389–402.

Werezak, L. and Stewart, N. (2002) 'Learning to live with early dementia.' *The Canadian Journal of Nursing Research 34*, 67–85.

Westburg, N. (1999) 'Hope in older women: The importance of past and current relationships.' *Adultspan Journal 1*(2), 79–90.

Wilkinson, K. (1996) 'The concept of hope in life-threatening illnesses.' *Professional Nurse 11*(10), 659–661.

Wolverson, E., Clarke, C. and Moniz-Cook, E. (2010) 'Remaining hopeful in early-stage dementia: A qualitative study.' *Aging and Mental Health 14*(4), 450–460.

Chapter 5

HUMOUR AND DEMENTIA

Chris Clarke and Helen Irwin

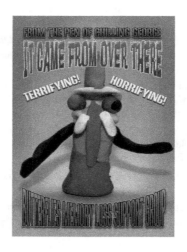

I think the next best thing to solving a problem is
finding some humor in it.

Frank A. Clark

A scientific solemnity usually surrounds dementia, and for good
reason, given the challenges and losses often associated with it. It would
be easy to assume that the experience of dementia therefore precludes
the ongoing personal expression or appreciation of humour. We may
be reluctant to consider a role for humour in the lives of people affected
by dementia for fear that they themselves could become objects of
mockery, thus perpetuating negative stereotypes and stigma. Equally,
it would neither be justifiable nor realistic to promote laughter and

humour if this did not concur with people's lived experiences and needs. We may simply ask: what is there to laugh about in dementia?

At the same time, many people living with or affected by dementia attest to the presence and importance of playfulness, laughter, joking and amusement in the context of having to deal with very serious challenges brought about by the condition (e.g. see Grierson, 2008). The preface to a book of jokes recently compiled by a group of people living with or affected by dementia neatly highlights this: 'This may seem an odd topic to address, as dementia is not viewed as a laughing matter by those affected by it. On the other hand, paradoxically, humour can be a very powerful means of coping in difficult circumstances' (Scottish Dementia Working Group, 2010, p.11).

Whilst exploring links between humour and dementia might therefore appear contradictory or even controversial, to refute the meaningful significance of humour and laughter in the lives of people living with dementia, however they occur, would risk denying important aspects of people's lived experiences. Humour is part of these experiences and relates directly to aspects of identity, coping and positive well-being.

Accordingly, this chapter aims to highlight the role and potential value of humour in the subjective experiences of people living with dementia. We start with an overview of the nature and function of humour and, pertinently, its relation to physical and psychological well-being and close relationships. The potential for humour to play a significant role in adjusting positively to living with a health condition is also discussed with reference to existing research in this area. We then consider how the experience of humour may alter as we age, before exploring the nascent literature on humour in dementia. As an illustration of the presence and potential value of humour in dementia, we describe the main findings of a qualitative study we conducted that explored the co-constructed meanings that humour may have for couples when one member of the dyad is experiencing dementia.

THE NATURE AND FUNCTIONS OF HUMOUR

Humour is a universal and fundamental aspect of being human but has different meanings and facets. It relates to what amuses us, how much we laugh or smile, how others make us laugh or smile or perhaps subtle combinations of all of these aspects. Martin (2007), perhaps the most prolific of humour researchers, conceptualises humour as a form of social communication that has evolved as a way of allowing people to engage in mental and social play. This form of social playfulness brings benefits in terms of positive emotions, strengthened relationships and greater social cohesiveness.

The appreciation of humour requires a playful mode of thinking and relating, where we recognise and then resolve some kind of incongruity in what is being said or shown to us or what we are experiencing. To do this, we playfully enjoy the apparent contradiction between different ideas as well as the disconfirmation of our expectations (Apter, 1982). Humour therefore involves the emotion of surprise as an incongruity or contradiction is realised and resolved (see Weems, 2014). Our experience of mirth – the pleasurable emotional state resulting from humour (Martin, 2007) – can depend on the nature of humorous stimuli (e.g. incongruity, timing and punch lines of jokes), our moods and, importantly in this context, whether our circumstances and social environments are conducive to playfulness and fun (i.e. safe and inclusive). The typical behavioural expression of humour is in the form of laughter. Whilst humour and laughter usually co-occur, they are not synonymous; we may not always laugh at what we find funny or amusing and, conversely, we may laugh in the absence of humour.

Sense of humour is a term used to describe individual differences in humour at a trait-level. Yet, this term may also have different meanings and connotations and, again, social contexts are likely to shape how a person's sense of humour is expressed. Sense of humour may be understood as a stable pattern of behaviour, a habitual way of coping, a temperamental style (e.g. trait cheerfulness; see Ruch and Carrell, 1998) or even an enduring set of positive and humorous attitudes. Martin (2007, p.195) describes sense of humour as 'a group of traits and abilities having to do with different components, forms and functions of humour [some of which] may be closely related…while others are likely to be quite distinct'.

From a positive psychology perspective, sense of humour can be conceptualised as a character strength – an acquired set of knowledge and skills that permit the display of a certain positive virtue (Peterson and Seligman, 2004). Character strengths are considered to be morally desirable, dimensional (i.e. varying between people), stable across time and circumstances, and cultivated through life-span development. In the classificatory framework of strengths known as

Values in Action (VIA), Peterson and Park (2004, p.438) frame humour in terms of playfulness, that is, 'liking to laugh and tease; bringing smiles to other people; seeing the light side; making (not necessarily telling) jokes'. Humour is further seen as one manifestation of the psychological virtue of transcendence – the ability to 'forge connections to the larger universe and provide meaning'. This framework allows for the possibility that, for some people, humour and playfulness are 'signature' strengths that nourish well-being even in the face of adversity. Humour has also been linked with hopefulness (see Vilaythong *et al.*, 2003), itself another character strength representative of the virtue of transcendence, according to the VIA framework.

As a trait-like character strength, humour is framed unidimensionally. However, the use of humour can be positive and negative, and varies according to whether it is focused on others or oneself. Martin and colleagues have therefore distinguished between four *styles* of humour:

- *Affiliative humour* is the tendency to use humour positively to amuse people and enhance interpersonal relationships.

- *Aggressive humour* refers to the tendency to employ humour negatively towards others as a means to mock, deride or criticise.

- *Self-enhancing humour* refers to the tendency to maintain a humorous approach to life, even when encountering adversity, in order to cope and preserve well-being.

- *Self-defeating humour* involves using humour negatively at one's own expense, perhaps as a way to avoid negative feelings whilst seeking social approval.

An important function of humour relates to how it helps maintain and enhance close relationships. Humour is related to greater perceived social support and higher quality of social relationships (for an overview, see Martin, 2007). Humour may serve different positive functions in close relationships: it can enhance intimacy and bonding but also help diffuse tension and manage conflict (see Butzer and Kuiper, 2008). Positive humour styles (affiliative and self-enhancing) are also associated with other pro-social factors, such as empathy (see Hampes, 2010).

HUMOUR AND HEALTH

The potential value of exploring humour in relation to dementia might be illustrated by first exploring links between humour, health and ageing more generally. A link between humour and good health has long been assumed but only researched relatively recently. To date, research findings in this area indicate that humour might have beneficial effects, albeit not as consistently as might be expected.

PSYCHOLOGICAL HEALTH

Research has indicated that humour generally tends to be positively associated with self-esteem, optimism and positive emotion (see Martin, 2007). Other research findings highlight that the impact of humour on well-being depends on the relative presence and absence of positive and negative styles. Self-enhancing and affiliative humour styles in particular have been found to be positively associated with a range of well-being measures and negatively associated with levels of anxiety and depression. In contrast, aggressive and self-defeating humour styles have been associated with lowered relationship satisfaction and increased levels of anxiety and depression, respectively (see Martin *et al.*, 2003).

Such associations have lent weight to the notion that humour acts as a moderator (or buffer) against stress. In general, studies investigating this have indicated that people who score highly on measures of humour tend to display lower signs of stress in response to life events than do people who score lower on such measures. In addition, there is evidence that humour moderates the impact of positive and negative life events on positive mood and well-being over time, boosting the impact of positive events whilst dampening the impact of the negative (see Martin *et al.*, 1993). Positive forms of humour may be protective against stress because they involve adaptive cognitive and behavioural coping strategies. For example, some research evidence indicates that higher levels of humour are linked with the tendency to perceive negative experiences as challenging rather threatening (e.g. see Kuiper, McKenzie and Belanger, 1995). At the behavioural level, humour has been associated with coping responses aimed at regulating emotions, confronting sources of stress and taking a philosophical, accepting approach to adversity (for an overview, see Martin, 2007).

PHYSICAL HEALTH

It is often said that 'laughter is the best medicine' but given that humour itself is multi-faceted and complex, any impact or association it may have on or with health and illness is unlikely to be straightforward and could involve different mechanisms. Humour could have direct beneficial effects on health through the physiological effects of laughter and mirth – by way of positive effects on immunological and cardiovascular functioning, for example. Alternatively, humour may moderate the impact of stress on health and illness primarily because it promotes perspective taking and challenge-based appraisals. Another potential mechanism is that humour is beneficial for health because it is associated with better social support and higher-quality social relationships (see earlier), which enhance health and improve adjustment to illness.

It is possible that these mechanisms occur in parallel or apply to certain aspects of health and illness (see Martin and Lefcourt, 2004). Some evidence indicates that humour provides a buffer against the impact of illness symptoms in a similar way to its ability to moderate the impact of stressful life events on psychological health (e.g. Carver *et al.*, 1993). As already noted, the way in which humour is used in relationships also impacts on its potential to beneficially affect well-being and this is of relevance to the role of humour in illness. Manne and colleagues (2004), for example, investigated the use of humour in self-disclosure interactions between women being treated for breast cancer and their spouses. They found that the use of benign humour by partners in response to the disclosure of cancer-concerns and problems contributed to lower levels of cancer-related distress amongst the patients (see Martin, 2007). This suggests that certain kinds of humour can have an effect on aspects of health as they interact with elements of close relationships, perhaps through the strengthening of intimacy or enhancement of shared problem solving.

The potential for humour to play a multi-dimensional role for people coping with a serious and chronic illness has been illustrated by qualitative studies exploring how humour is used and perceived in cancer. Rose, Spencer and Rausch (2013), for example, conducted a phenomenological study of the meanings and uses of humour amongst 17 women receiving treatment for recurrent ovarian cancer. Key themes to emerge across interviews included positive appraisals of the use of humour, the need to build trust with health professionals before humour was considered useful, and humour being informal and tied in with everyday anecdotes rather than specific jokes and the perceived need for humour prior to consultations with health professionals. The authors frame humour in this context as an important self-enhancing coping strategy rather than a form of avoidance. Similar findings and interpretations were reported by Chapple and Ziebland (2004), who conducted a qualitative study of humour use amongst 45 men diagnosed with testicular cancer. In this group, humour was also cast as an important coping strategy that had a variety of functions in relation to coping with the impact of cancer and surgery. Of potential relevance to dementia, the authors suggest that in health conditions the use of humour becomes 'applied' to the social realm in order to convey 'serious' concerns and manage power imbalances in relationships (e.g. with health professionals).

HUMOUR IN AGEING

Humour is widely recognised for its beneficial effects on physiological and psychological health across the life-span (e.g. Pressman and Cohen, 2005). Fry (1986) proposed that humour is a health-promoting behaviour essential to successful ageing. Despite this, most prominent definitions of successful ageing, the majority of which have been derived from theoretical literature, do not include humour. Arguably, however, such definitions should be based on the values of older people themselves. Research indicates that older people incorporate having a sense of humour into their views of successful ageing (see Guse and Masesar, 1999; Tate, Lah and Cuddy, 2003). Lurie and Monahan (2015) draw attention to the multiple ways in which humour facilitates important factors and processes connected with well-being in ageing, including maintenance of self-worth and identity, successful life-review, coping with loss and overcoming fear of death. Because of these benefits, psychotherapeutic interventions aimed at eliciting and enhancing humour in late life have been subject to empirical study in recent years. Collectively, such research indicates that in later life 'humour therapies' are capable of improving quality of life and well-being and reducing anxiety and depression (Irwin, Clarke and Wolverson, 2015).

Whilst some studies have begun to shed light on the experience of humour in later life, it is difficult to draw firm conclusions from the literature because research has often been cross-sectional, comparing humour in older and younger adults, which makes it difficult to distinguish between age differences or cohort effects (Greengross, 2013). The lack of consensus within the literature may also reflect the various ways humour has been defined and measured. Some studies have attempted to measure humour production, comprehension and appreciation in older age. There is some evidence to suggest that the ability to produce and comprehend humour reduces in later life if there is a corresponding decline in cognitive ability (e.g. Mak and Carpenter, 2007). We might therefore assume that humour appreciation, defined as the enjoyment of a joke, would also decline. However, research findings generally suggest the contrary: humour appreciation actually increases with age. In line with incongruity accounts of humour (see earlier), age-related cognitive decline might make jokes more difficult to understand but it could also make them funnier because it is the sudden discovery of the point of the joke that is the source of humour. However, if cognitive impairment exceeds a certain level, a joke could place too much cognitive demand on the individual, restricting appreciation and enjoyment (e.g. Schaier and Cicirelli, 1976).

Yet humour involves much more than circumscribed jokes, and the ability to enjoy a joke could therefore be considered a crude measure of humour appreciation. Herth (1993) suggested that humour appreciation does not decline but rather the function and perception of humour changes. Factors such as changes in sensory perception and the occurrence of adverse life experiences (e.g. chronic illness, isolation and bereavement) in older age may influence this. However, more broadly, ageing has been associated with better emotion regulation and increased well-being in comparison to younger adult (Aldwin and Yancura, 2010). What positive resources are older adults drawing upon to achieve this? There is some evidence to suggest that older adults use humour more frequently as a coping strategy than younger adults and have a more positive outlook towards humour (e.g. Thorson and Powell, 1993). Herth (1993) hypothesised that an internal sense of humour becomes important rather than external sources of humour. This is supported by Martin (2007), who suggests that in later life humour is used more as a way of upholding a more humorous outlook on life (i.e. self-enhancing humour).

HUMOUR AND DEMENTIA

Literature highlighting the role and impact of humour in health and ageing prompts important questions pertinent to living with dementia. Do people with dementia express, appreciate and find benefit from humour? Does humour moderate the impact of dementia in certain ways? What role does humour play in close relationships in dementia? In seeking answers to these questions, however, we quickly encounter the problem that, in comparison with other health conditions and forms of disability, relatively little is known about humour in dementia and it has not, so far, attracted the attention it deserves from researchers and clinicians. This may be for two reasons. First, some have dissuaded the use of humour in the context of psychological distress and cognitive impairment, in the belief that it is ethically wrong and risks causing offence (e.g. Hunt, 1993). Second, it might easily be assumed that people with dementia do not have the cognitive capacity to partake in or genuinely appreciate humour. This might be seen as a reasonable assumption, given the literature suggesting that significantly impaired cognitive function hinders the ability to appreciate humour (Schaier and Cicirelli, 1976; Svebak, Martin and Jostein, 2004). Humour has often been regarded as a coping strategy and, as suggested by Dröes (2007), until recently it was assumed that people with dementia did not actively engage in coping strategies because of impaired self-awareness. However, an increasing number of studies and viewpoints have been steadily challenging such positions.

In recent years, there has been growing recognition and appreciation that people with dementia are, and should be recognised as, active agents in pursuit of well-being and positive identity. Kitwood and Bredin (1992) highlight the expression and appreciation of humour as an important indicator of positive well-being and personhood in living with dementia – indeed, anyone privileged enough to know or work with someone who lives with dementia would most likely endorse this. In support, Liptak and colleagues (2013) conducted a study in which instances of humour were coded in focus groups of people with mild cognitive impairment and Alzheimer's disease. They reported that humour and laughter were present in all of the focus group interviews and described the themes of humour as silliness, sarcasm and commenting about the difficulties of dementia, providing evidence that people with cognitive impairment can engage in humour and may use it as a coping mechanism (i.e. they may cope by laughing about dementia and its impact).

Overall, qualitative research suggests that humour could hold particular significance for people as an aspect of selfhood, a personal strength or coping resource as they actively engage in living with the condition (Wolverson, Clarke and Moniz-Cook, 2016; see also Chapter 2). Similarly, in a review of commonly occurring themes in the lived experience literature, Snyder (2001) draws attention to how important it is for the person with dementia and their caregivers to encourage and experience humour in their daily lives and for humour to be used socially as a way of bringing people together in a shared experience, rather than feeling isolated. The literature also suggests that people with dementia laugh at dementia-related symptoms – one man stated, whilst watching children hunt for Easter eggs, 'Now that I have Alzheimer's, I can hide my own Easter eggs' (p.19). People with dementia laughing at their own difficulties has been interpreted within the literature as a coping mechanism (Langdon, Eagle and Warner, 2006; Van Dijkhuizen, Clare and Pearce, 2006) and therefore a self-enhancing form of humour designed to maintain positive well-being. This form of humour might also act as a way of redressing power imbalances in social contexts that surround the experience of a disability (see Shakespeare, 1999).

The existence and benefits of humour may also extend into later 'stages' of dementia. Takeda *et al.* (2010) argue that whilst humour use in relation to social communication may be compromised to varying extents in the early stages of dementia, the beneficial effects of laughter in terms of promoting pleasant feelings and the release of tension can be maintained even in advanced dementia. In detailed case studies of three people described as living with severe Alzheimer's disease, Moos (2011) presents some evidence that the participants could express themselves with aspects of humour, including plays on words, irony and sarcasm, despite limited verbal and memory abilities. As Moos subsequently concludes, the use of humour by these participants represents a challenge to the notion of 'retrogenesis' in dementia, which assumes that cognitive and communicative abilities acquired later in childhood development are the first to be irretrievably lost as dementia progresses. In using aspects of humour within interpersonal interactions, her participants demonstrated a continued ability to understand and express the essence of humour and, in doing so, simultaneously expressed their desire to actively communicate their needs, personhood and autonomy.

Humour may play an important moderating role in caregiving relationships in dementia, adding further challenge to the assumption that its use is inappropriate. Caregivers report placing value on humour as a useful coping strategy to relieve stress and burden and as a way of uplifting spirits in the context of supporting a loved one with living with dementia (see Jathanna, Latha and Bhandary, 2010; Tan and Schneider, 2009). However, within the caregiver literature, the role of humour could also be an important component of the caregiving relationship. For example, in writing about their own personal experience of living with dementia, Dolores and Desmond Smith (2012) reported that laughter had always been an important part of their marriage and became even more crucial when Dolores developed Alzheimer's disease. The couple describe how humour 'promotes a sense of light heartedness that improves the state of mind' (p.7).

In line with current initiatives within health and social care – for example, the National Dementia Strategy for England (Department of Health, 2009) – towards promoting 'living well' and improving the quality of life of those with dementia, some studies have investigated the potential beneficial effect of humour interventions for people with dementia. Early research studies (e.g. Walter *et al.*, 2007) were limited by low sample sizes and did not show clear effects on quality of life. However, subsequent qualitative and quantitative studies have indicated that it is possible to involve people living with dementia in therapeutic humour programmes and that such programmes can have a positive impact on outcomes such as quality of life and even cognitive functioning. Stevens (2011) designed a humour programme for people with dementia living in the community, teaching them how to perform stand-up comedy over eight weekly sessions. The aim was to actively engage people with dementia in creating comedy and making themselves and others laugh. Qualitative data from semi-structured interviews with participants and their caregivers revealed perceived improvements in a variety of areas including memory, learning, social ability, communication and self-esteem.

In another participatory intervention study conducted by Hafford-Letchfield (2013), people with dementia took part in comedy workshops that were aimed at making a short mockumentary about 'Her Majesty the Queen' visiting the day centre, mainly using improvisation. The workshops were not evaluated using formal measures, but observations and reports from the people involved suggested that the workshops provided enjoyment for the participants, and improved mood, alertness and concentration. Increased well-being and reduced stress levels were reported in family caregivers, and observations also indicated that the workshops improved relationships and communication between participants, family caregivers and staff members.

Such effects were echoed in the findings of a recent randomised controlled trial. Conducted by Low and colleagues (2013), this study investigated the impact of humour therapy in 189 nursing home residents, the majority of whom were living with dementia. One staff member from each nursing home was given training on practical ways to encourage humour in daily care. The intervention also consisted of personalised interactions (e.g. songs, games, dance and jokes) to encourage fun and laughter for participants. Following the humour therapy, the participants in the intervention group showed a significant reduction in agitation and a significant improvement in quality of life and social engagement.

Whilst humour is therefore present in dementia and in caregiving relationships, and some evidence indicates that it can be nurtured and enhanced to improve well-being and quality of life, there remain important questions about how people experience the positive effects of humour in living with dementia and how humour operates in close relationships in dementia. The latter issue is particularly important, given that the active use of humour in close relationships may be a key way in which humour acts as a positive buffer against the impact of a chronic health condition in one member of the dyad. In dementia, this takes on further potential importance as couples seek to accept and make sense of the condition together, whilst also striving to maintain their sense of couplehood (see Merrick, Camic and O'Shaughnessy, 2013). In our own research work, we have explored these issues by taking a lived experience and relational perspective on the use of humour in couples where one person is living with dementia.

SHARED EXPERIENCES OF HUMOUR IN DEMENTIA: KEY FINDINGS FROM A QUALITATIVE STUDY

We conducted an exploratory study (see Irwin, Wolverson and Clarke, 2015) to investigate how people with dementia and their partners use, experience and draw meaning from humour in their ongoing relationships. Semi-structured interviews were used with ten couples in order to explore subjective experiences of humour in relationships before and after diagnosis of dementia as well as the perceived role of humour in relationships in the context of everyday life with dementia. Interviews were transcribed in full and analysed using Interpretative Phenomenological Analysis (Smith, Flowers and Larkin, 1999). This process led to the identification of three superordinate and eight sub-themes concerning the role, meaning and functions of humour for couples living with dementia (see Table 5.1).

Table 5.1: Master table of themes from a qualitative study of humour in dementia

SUPERORDINATE THEME	SUB-THEME
Humour has always been there and always will be	Humour comes naturally
	Still laughing
Dementia is a threat to humour	Coming to terms with the diagnosis of dementia
	Changing abilities of the person with dementia
	Changing lifestyle
Humour is important in living with dementia	Realising the value of humour
	Making light of the situation
	Increasing positive emotions

For the purposes of this chapter, case studies of three of the couples who took part in this research will be presented and used to illustrate a selection of the above themes.

Couple 1: Angela and Dave

Angela and Dave had been together for 36 years at the time of participating in the research. Angela had received a diagnosis of Alzheimer's disease four years previously. They readily reported that humour had always played a significant part in their relationship and continues to do so, in spite of Angela's dementia. There was a sense that humour had evolved throughout their relationship and with age, in order to meet their changing needs as a couple. For this reason, humour was viewed as a private experience between them, not necessarily something that other people would understand:

> **Dave:** We have a good laugh and we do have some funny times… It's like personal and private, that's when your humour comes in, 'cos we can say things and do things, without offending people, we find humorous but other people wouldn't appreciate.

In their relationship, Dave had always been the initiator of humour and this had not changed in the context of living with dementia:

> **Dave:** I make the jokes! [laughs]

> **Angela:** I know you've got a joke in your pocket somewhere!

However, the couple explained that shared humour was becoming increasingly more difficult as Angela's increasing cognitive impairment meant that she was finding it more difficult to understand and appreciate the sense of humour they had previously shared:

> **Dave:** That's one of the sad things about the illness, all that stuff goes, humour and…'cos you need [points to head] to pick up on things.

Despite the threat that dementia posed to humour, Dave and Angela described how important humour was in living with dementia in terms of changing perspective and fostering positive feelings. As Angela's dementia progressed, Dave adapted his humour style to Angela's abilities in order to maintain humour in their relationship:

> **Dave:** Yeah so it's changed, it has changed, it's still important, but, more important really but it's not so... instantaneous because I haven't that feedback with words and dialogue, you know a conversation when I can turn things on their head or move them around a bit you know, that's that...missing, so it's a bit, it's changed a lot, so I clown about more now, yeah.

Dave spoke about how sometimes it was difficult to maintain a sense of humour because the stress and fatigue associated with caregiving had a negative impact on his humour:

> **Dave:** We get depressed, demoralised, demotivated, all this comes in and it's difficult to keep pulling yourself up and keep going... It all impinges on our everyday lives [and] humour.

Yet humour was vital in helping him cope with and relieve the negative emotions of caregiving:

> **Dave:** It's a release; it's breaking the frustration, the tension, the aggravation, the anger...

For this couple dementia posed a very real threat to humour but they were working actively to adapt, change and maintain their humour, because, for them, humour played a significant part in their relationship and living with dementia.

Couple 2: Raymond and Sheila

Raymond and Sheila had been together for 42 years at the time of participating in the study. Raymond had received a diagnosis of Alzheimer's disease seven months previously.

Raymond and Sheila also described the value of humour in their relationship in living with dementia:

Raymond: I don't think it's [humour] changed but it's become more important.

Sheila: Mmm, yeah, 'cos we do go down at times you know [coughs] and we come back up again, yeah.

In contrast to Dave and Angela, who had clearly reflected on the importance of humour within their relationship and coping with dementia prior to the interview, Raymond and Sheila seemed only to realise its value when prompted to think about it in the interview:

Raymond: I never realised how important it was, but now I do. I've had a reason to try and analyse it and see what benefit it is.

Raymond and Sheila also described dementia as a threat to humour, but in a different way to Dave and Angela. They described coming to terms with the diagnosis of dementia as the threat to humour. Several other couples also described how the process of coming to terms with a diagnosis of dementia was a particularly difficult and challenging time, accompanied by negative emotions such as shock and worry. Because of these overriding negative emotions, humour was less present:

Sheila: There's not been so much [humour] there because it was a big shock you know and we are still coming to terms with it.

However, at the same time, humour helped this couple, and several others, cope with and adjust to the diagnosis. Sheila felt that at this time humour was especially important, and together they actively used humour in order to help them come to terms with the diagnosis, as humour functioned as a way of coping with the accompanying negative emotions. Humour was still present even during these difficult times post-diagnosis:

Sheila: We are still coming to terms with it but I mean we still do try and laugh at things you know because you have to, you know, otherwise you would go barmy wouldn't you?

For Sheila and Raymond humour was used as a mechanism to help them live in and enjoy the present moment instead of worrying about the future, in particular the future prognosis of dementia:

> **Raymond:** It makes you come to terms with the presence [sic] because it's so much in the presence [sic] I certainly see it as a positive aspect, one of the few positive aspects that I can come up with at the moment [laughs]...but if it changes me perspective, our perspective, I think on that then that will be good for us.

> **Raymond:** Whatever worries you may have, they disappear with humour don't they?

For Raymond, humour was also an important tool to help him to communicate with others and he describes why this has been especially important since his diagnosis of dementia:

> **Raymond:** ...I think humour is increasingly becoming more and more important...memory's a funny thing... it affects all sorts of things but it doesn't affect the one-liner. As a one-liner, the humorous one-liner is useful in all sorts of situations, particularly social; it reduces tension, makes you relax, so making other people laugh is...is more, is increasingly more important to me. I'm finding it's a way of communicating as well. It breaks down barriers etc. so I've noticed, you know, specifically that it is definitely more important now... So everything about humour is positive.

Couple 3: Val and Roy

Val and Roy had been together for 53 years at the time of the study. Val had been diagnosed with vascular dementia four years previously. For Val and Roy, humour was an integral part of their daily lives and relationship, past and present. They described using humour 'every hour of every day' and this was evident in their interview as they shared humorous stories and jokes and laughed throughout:

Val: Oh, we don't stop laughing! [Both then laugh]

Humour had been used by Val and Roy equally throughout their relationship as a coping strategy in the face of adversity, in part as a way of making light of the situation, and in part because laughter simply lifted their mood:

Val: We don't really take anything serious do we?

Roy: No.

Roy: It's the best medicine is laughter.

Val: It is!

They explained that humour had become more salient since the diagnosis of dementia and they recognised that this was because humour was a useful coping strategy in managing the difficulties faced when living with dementia. They used humour to make light of an otherwise overwhelming or upsetting situation, and for them there was a corresponding sense that dementia would be too difficult to manage without humour:

Val: It [dementia] would be too heavy wouldn't it?

Roy: Oh I think it is, yeah. When you think of some of the pressure that could be on you, you know, like they all say, what was mentioned ten minutes ago or maybe just before you came in, if you don't see the funny side you'll cry, or you could cry over some of the, you know, sort of personal things.

Several couples described how humour helped them cope with the difficulties posed by dementia. However, it was also that humour was not just a coping strategy in response to dementia. For some, humour was a way of life, and this was particularly demonstrated by Val and Roy. As such, they brought their humour to bear on dementia itself. They humorously related a story of when Val had gone to get some eggs from their neighbour whilst Roy had waited for her in the car. Half an hour later, Val returned to Roy without the eggs only to realise that she had been standing at their neighbour's door for half an hour, without knocking, wondering what she had gone there for in the first place. Whilst ostensibly an anecdote about the frustrations of living with dementia, both Val and Roy had identified this situation as a source of genuine and shared humour, and laughed together whilst relating their story about it. This is particularly noteworthy because of the way that Val and Roy jointly turned humour upon dementia itself; together they succeed in what Shakespeare (1999, p.51) calls a 'reversal of expectation [which] is always richly comedic, and there is no greater reversal than treating what is commonly represented as a tragedy as if it is a farce'. In doing so, they took control over impairment whilst strengthening their bond as a couple.

CONCLUSIONS

If we consider the findings of this study alongside the broader literature on humour in illness, disability and ageing reviewed in this chapter, a number of key issues about the possible role of humour in dementia can be distilled. Humour, in varying forms, is not just present in the lives of people with dementia but carries significant meanings and functions as a buffer against the impact of dementia, enabling a sense of safety and the experience of positive emotion that is known to be linked with positive health more generally. This may occur directly through the experience of mirth or indirectly through humour-related perspective-taking, but it is also likely that the positive effects of humour only occur within the context of positive relationships and meaningful conversations.

Some people living with dementia are likely to have used and enjoyed humour all of their lives. Their sense of humour, expressed in varying ways, may represent an important character strength in relation to playfulness and the capacity for transcendence, possibly facilitating the ability to go 'beyond' immediate adversity and maintain deeper connections with loved ones and the world in general. We need to know more about how individual differences in humour styles impact on well-being and relationships in dementia. The extent to which cognitive impairment really does change the appreciation of incongruities, irony and playfulness in more advanced dementia is also an important area of further inquiry. Both qualitative and quantitative research methods should be brought to bear on such topics (see Lockyer, 2006) but this should, above all, be a collaborative inquiry with people living with dementia themselves.

Similar to those experiencing a physical health condition, people living with dementia might also use humour *about* dementia, not merely to ease tension or gain acceptance but to maintain identity, re-assert a sense of control and, ultimately, to challenge social stereotypes and taboos. As Shakespeare (1999) warns, making jokes out of any form of disability runs a fine line between reinforcing stereotypes and subverting them. The risk of inadvertently making light of dementia is a significant one in terms of invalidating the full range of people's experiences, and we certainly do not advocate a light-hearted approach to humour in dementia here. Much depends on the contexts in which the humour is being created, who is generating it and what or whom exactly is being laughed at. On the one hand, people with dementia are vulnerable to being passive recipients of aggressive forms of joking and laughter on a societal level, replete with nihilistic and 'othering' narratives about dementia as loss of mind and self, but also by often well-intentioned care-partners (Kitwood, 1997). On the other hand, close supportive relationships involving trust and empathy are likely to be key to an experience of humour that is affiliative and self-enhancing and that, in turn, positively impacts the quality of such relationships and their potential for upholding personhood. More broadly, as the studies by Stevens (2011) and Hafford-Letchfield (2013) illustrate, in the right social environment, people with dementia can be empowered to take the lead on generating humour. That a book of jokes has been compiled and produced by a group of people living with dementia is another important illustration of how people can claim their right to humour (Scottish Dementia Working Group, 2010). Doing so represents a powerful way to reverse expectation on a social level and so challenge and change assumptions about living with dementia.

REFERENCES

Aldwin, C. and Yancura, L. (2010) 'Effects of stress on health and aging: Two paradoxes.' *California Agriculture* 64(4), 183–188.

Apter, M.J. (1982) *The Experience of Motivation: The Theory of Psychological Reversals.* London: Academic Press.

Butzer, B. and Kuiper, N.A. (2008) 'Humor use in romantic relationships: The effects of relationship satisfaction and pleasant versus conflict situations.' *The Journal of Psychology 142*(3), 245–260.

Carver, C.S., Pozo, C., Harris, S.D., Noriega, V. *et al.* (1993) 'How coping mediates the effect of optimism on distress: A study of women with early stage breast cancer.' *Journal of Personality and Social Psychology 65*(2), 375.

Chapple, A. and Ziebland, S. (2004) 'The role of humor for men with testicular cancer.' *Qualitative Health Research 14*(8), 1123–1139.

Department of Health (2009) *Living well with dementia: A national dementia strategy.* Available at: www.gov.uk/government/publications/living-well-with-dementia-a-national-dementia-strategy, accessed on 15 Nov 2015.

Dröes, R.M. (2007) 'Insight in coping with dementia: Listening to the voice of those who suffer from it.' *Aging and Mental Health 11*(2), 115–118.

Fry, W. (1986) 'Humor, Physiology, and Aging Process.' In L. Nahemow, K. McCluskey-Fawcett and P. McGhee (eds) *Humor and Aging.* Orlando, FL: Academic Press.

Greengross, G. (2013) 'Humor and aging – a mini-review.' *Gerontology 59*(5), 448–453.

Grierson, J. (2008) *Knickers in the Fridge.* Great Britain: Lulu.

Guse, L.W. and Masesar, M.A. (1999) 'Quality of life and successful aging in long-term care: Perceptions of residents.' *Issues in Mental Health Nursing 20*(6), 527–539.

Hafford-Letchfield, T. (2013) 'Funny things happen at the Grange: Introducing comedy activities in day services to older people with dementia: Innovative practice.' *Dementia 12*(6), 840–852.

Hampes, W.P. (2010) 'The relation between humor styles and empathy.' *Europe's Journal of Psychology 6*(3), 34–45.

Herth, K.A. (1993) 'Humor and the older adult.' *Applied Nursing Research 6*(4), 146–153.

Hunt, A.H. (1993) 'Humor as a nursing intervention.' *Cancer Nursing 16*(1), 34–39.

Irwin. H., Clarke. C. and Wolverson. E. (2015) *The impact of humour interventions on physical and psychological wellbeing in later life: A systematic literature review.* Unpublished doctoral thesis, University of Hull, Hull.

Irwin, H., Wolverson, E. and Clarke, C. (2015). Humour and dementia – a qualitative study of the shared experience of humour between people living with dementia and their partners. Unpublished doctoral thesis, University of Hull, Hull.

Jathanna, R.P., Latha K.S., L. and Bhandary, P.V. (2011) 'Burden and coping in informal caregivers of persons with dementia: A cross sectional study.' *Online Journal of Health and Allied Sciences 9*(4) 1–6.

Kitwood, T. (1997) *Dementia Reconsidered.* Buckingham: Open University Press.

Kitwood, T. and Bredin, K. (1992) 'Towards a theory of dementia care: Personhood and well-being.' *Ageing and Society 12*(3), 269–287.

Langdon, S.A., Eagle, A. and Warner, J. (2007) 'Making sense of dementia in the social world: A qualitative study.' *Social Science and Medicine 64*(4), 989–1000.

Liptak, A., Tate, J., Flatt, J., Oakley, M.A. and Lingler, J. (2013) 'Humor and laughter in persons with cognitive impairment and their caregivers.' *Journal of Holistic Nursing 32*(1), 25–34.

Lockyer, S. (2006) 'Heard the one about...applying mixed methods in humour research?' *International Journal of Social Research Methodology 9*(1), 41–59.

Low, L.F., Brodaty, H., Goodenough, B., Spitzer, P. *et al.* (2013) 'The Sydney Multisite Intervention of LaughterBosses and ElderClowns (SMILE) study: Cluster randomised trial of humour therapy in nursing homes.' *BMJ Open 3*(1), e002072.

Lurie, A. and Monahan, K. (2015) 'Humor, aging, and life review: Survival through the use of humor.' *Social Work in Mental Health 13*(1), 82–91.

Mak, W. and Carpenter, B.D. (2007) 'Humor comprehension in older adults.' *Journal of the International Neuropsychological Society 13*(4), 606–614.

Manne, S., Sherman, M., Ross, S., Ostroff, J., Heyman, R.E. and Fox, K. (2004) 'Couples' support-related communication, psychological distress, and relationship satisfaction among women with early stage breast cancer.' *Journal of Consulting and Clinical Psychology 72*(4), 660.

Martin, R.A. (2007) *The Psychology of Humor: An Integrative Approach.* Burlington, MA: Elsevier Academic Press.

Martin, R.A., Kuiper, N.A., Olinger, L.J. and Dance, K.A. (1993) 'Humor, coping with stress, self-concept, and psychological well-being.' *Humor 6*, 89–104.

Martin, R.A. and Lefcourt, H.M. (2004) 'Sense of humor and physical health: Theoretical issues, recent findings, and future directions.' *Humor 17*(1–2), 1–20.

Martin, R.A., Puhlik-Doris, P., Larsen, G., Gray, J. and Weir, K. (2003) 'Individual differences in uses of humor and their relation to psychological well-being: Development of the Humor Styles Questionnaire.' *Journal of Research in Personality 37*(1), 48–75.

Merrick, K., Camic, P.M. and O'Shaughnessy, M. (2013) 'Couples constructing their experiences of dementia: A relational perspective.' *Dementia.* DOI:1471301213513029

Moos, I. (2011) 'Humour, irony and sarcasm in severe Alzheimer's dementia – a corrective to retrogenesis?' *Ageing and Society 31*(2), 328–346.

Peterson, C. and Park, N. (2004) 'Classification and Measurement of Character Strengths: Implications for Practice.' In P.A. Linley and S. Joseph (eds) *Positive Psychology in Practice.* Hoboken, NJ: Wiley.

Peterson, C. and Seligman, M.E.P. (2004) *Character Strengths and Virtues: A Handbook of Classification.* New York, NY: Oxford University Press.

Pressman, S.D. and Cohen, S. (2005) 'Does positive affect influence health?' *Psychological Bulletin 131*(6), 925–971.

Rose, S.L., Spencer, R.J. and Rausch, M.M. (2013) 'The use of humor in patients with recurrent ovarian cancer: a phenomenological study.' *International Journal of Gynecological Cancer 23*(4), 775–779.

Ruch, W. and Carrell, A. (1998) 'Trait cheerfulness and the sense of humour.' *Personality and Individual Differences 24*(4), 551–558.

Schaier, A. H. and Cicirelli, V.G. (1976) 'Age differences in humor comprehension and appreciation in old age.' *Journal of Gerontology 31*(5), 577–582.

Scottish Dementia Working Group (2010) *Why Am I Laughing?* Glasgow: Waverley Books.

Shakespeare, T. (1999) 'Joking a part.' *Body and Society 5*(4), 47–52.

Smith, D. and Smith, D. (2012) 'Our journey with Alzheimer's disease.' *New Zealand Journal of Occupational Therapy 59*(2), 5–8.

Smith, J.A., Flowers, P. and Larkin, M. (2009) *Interpretive Phenomenological Analysis: Theory, Method and Research.* London: SAGE Publications Ltd.

Snyder, L. (2001) 'The lived experience of Alzheimer's – understanding the feelings and subjective accounts of persons with the disease.' *Alzheimer's Care Today 2*(2), 8–22.

Stevens, J. (2011) 'Stand up for dementia: Performance, improvisation and stand up comedy as therapy for people with dementia: A qualitative study.' *Dementia, 11*(1), 61–73.

Svebak, S., Martin, R.A. and Jostein. H. (2004) 'The prevalence of sense of humor in a large, unselected county population in Norway: Relations with age, sex, and some health indicators.' *Humor 17*(1–2), 121–134.

Takeda, M., Hashimoto, R., Kudo, T., Okochi, M. *et al.* (2010) 'Laughter and humor as complementary and alternative medicines for dementia patients.' *BMC Complementary and Alternative Medicine 10*(1), 10–28.

Tan, T. and Schneider, M.A. (2009) 'Humor as a coping strategy for adult–child caregivers of individuals with Alzheimer's disease.' *Geriatric Nursing 30*(6), 397–408.

Tate, R.B., Lah, L. and Cuddy, T.E. (2003) 'Definition of successful aging by elderly Canadian males: The Manitoba follow-up study.' *The Gerontologist 43*(5), 735–744.

Thorson, J.A. and Powell, F.C. (1993) 'Sense of humor and dimensions of personality.' *Journal of Clinical Psychology 49*(6), 799–809.

Van Dijkhuizen, M., Clare, L. and Pearce, A. (2006) 'Striving for connection: Appraisal and coping among women with early-stage Alzheimer's disease.' *Dementia 5*(1), 73–94.

Vilaythong, A.P., Arnau, R.C., Rosen, D.H. and Mascaro, N. (2003) 'Humor and hope: Can humor increase hope?' *Humor 16*(1), 79–90.

Walter, M., Hänni, B., Haug, M., Amrhein, I. *et al.* (2007) 'Humour therapy in patients with late-life depression or Alzheimer's disease: A pilot study.' *International Journal of Geriatric Psychiatry 22*(1), 77–83.

Wolverson, E.L., Clarke, C. and Moniz-Cook, E.D. (2016) 'Living positively with dementia: A systematic review and synthesis of the qualitative literature.' *Aging and Mental Health 20*(7): 676–699.

Weems, S. (2014) *Ha!: The Science of When We Laugh and Why.* Philadephia, PA: Perseus Books Group.

Chapter 6

RESILIENCE AND LIVING WELL WITH DEMENTIA

Phyllis Braudy Harris

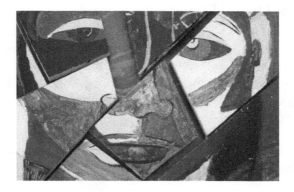

Dementia is the only disease or condition and the only terminal illness that I know of where patients are told to go home and give up their pre-diagnosis lives, rather than to 'fight for their lives.'

Kate Swaffer, a person living well with dementia (Swaffer, 2015, p.3)

Identifying and providing strategies that can maintain personal strengths and empower people to live well with dementia and remain contributing members of society for as long as possible are important priorities for us all. The concept of resilience may afford us some clues as to how this might be achieved, and the central aim of this chapter is to highlight how a resilience framework is potentially highly applicable to understanding how people might live well with dementia.

In pursuit of this, the chapter begins with a discussion of the concept of resilience in relation to life-span development and ageing, locating it historically as an alternative to the successful ageing movement. The chapter then explores how resilience might be involved in adapting to health conditions in later life, and in so doing how we can begin to discern its potential relevance to living with dementia. Within this context, the results of a qualitative study of the experience of resilience in early-stage dementia are then presented in order to demonstrate how, by using a resilience framework, positive promoting factors can be identified that might assist people to live well with dementia. The practice implications for clinicians of a resilience-focused perspective on living well with dementia are then presented and discussed.

SUCCESSFUL AGEING

In the early 1980s a paradigm shift occurred in gerontological research, turning the focus from the problems of ageing towards positive ageing. Much energy and resources since then have been devoted to defining and discovering the variables that affect so-called 'successful ageing' (i.e. those that help people to preserve and maintain physical and psychological well-being in later life). The landmark MacArthur Foundation Study of Successful Ageing by Rowe and Kahn (1998) fuelled this research. The Rowe and Kahn Health Promotion Model stresses that avoiding disease and disability, maintaining high mental and physical functioning and remaining socially engaged are all key to ageing successfully (see Rowe and Kahn, 1997). There were a number of other models: Baltes and Baltes' adaptation model of Selective Optimisation with Compensation (1990) describes adaptive behaviours that are initiated when the ratio of the losses over gains involved in ageing become disproportionate; the Vaillant Positive Ageing Model (see Vaillant, 2004) stresses the protective value of health promotion behaviours; and the Kahana and Kahana Preventive and Corrective Proactivity Model (1996, 2003), based on a stress-coping paradigm, considers adaptations and events that have occurred throughout the life course and their impact on ageing well. What these models have in common is their emphasis on prevention and individually modifiable health promotion behaviours that have the potential to preserve physical and psychological well-being in later life.

However, from the beginning, the term 'successful ageing' has been a controversial concept, and difficult to define and measure. It is also an exclusive concept, focused largely on objective health status and neither encompassing disability and disease nor acknowledging the structural and social factors that create disparities and social inequalities that influence the ageing process (Holstein and Minkler, 2003). Katz and Calasanti (2015) suggest that the concept of successful ageing is more appealing than illuminating because of its emphasis on factors that place success versus failure in ageing solely in the hands of the individual. This ignores the powerful impact of the social determinants of health: income, social class, gender, race and ethnicity, and environment. Such a stance excludes people who, by definition, cannot age 'successfully', including those with disabilities.

The concept of resilience provides an alternative perspective to successful ageing (see Martinson and Berridge, 2015). Given the reality of health challenges and social inequalities in later life, perhaps the true quest for ageing well should not be defined by successful ageing but should lie in fostering and maintaining resilience. This concept until recently was undervalued and not fully examined within the ageing literature. However, developing and maintaining resilience is possible for many older adults regardless of social and cultural backgrounds or physical and cognitive impairments (Harris, 2008).

RESILIENCE FRAMEWORK AND MEASUREMENT

Resilience is a concept that has multiple dimensions: psychological, physiological, emotional, spiritual, social and environmental (Allen *et al.*, 2011; Wild, Wiles and Allen, 2013). It might be more clearly conceptualised in terms of a 'resilience repertoire', a supply of skills and resources, which can help moderate or buffer adversities that one experiences in life in order to maintain well-being (Clark *et al.*, 2011; Hardy, Concato and Gill, 2002). Historically, there have been two differing viewpoints in the literature on resilience. One perspective defines resilience as a personality trait or individual characteristic of having the ability to successfully cope with misfortune (see Richardson, 2002). The other, now more common, perspective defines resilience as a dynamic, psycho-social process of positive adaptation, involving the use of positive coping strategies. Hence it is a behaviour (not a fixed trait), which can be learned or developed (Allen *et al.*, 2011; Luthar,

Cicchetti and Becker, 2000; Masten, 2001). Perhaps Windle (2012, p.159) best summarises this more accepted perspective:

> Resilience is the process of negotiating, managing and adapting to different sources of stress or trauma. Assets and resources within the individual, their life and environment facilitate this capacity for adaption and 'bouncing back'. This definition acknowledges key features of resilience: 1) the encounter with adversity, such as ill health, 2) the ability to resist, manage and adapt to adversity (drawing on resources), and 3) the maintenance of good mental health.

Research into resilience originally took a developmental approach and focused on children and adolescents. One of the goals of this research was to identify protective factors that assisted some children in surviving, adapting and thriving under adverse conditions (e.g. socio-economic disadvantages, parental mental illness, abuse and catastrophic life events) compared to others who did not (Cicchetti *et al.*, 2000; Luthar, 1999; Luthar and Zelazo, 2003; Masten and Coatsworth, 1998). Examples of some of those protective factors fell into three key categories: *individual*, such as positive view of self, secure attachment in infancy, positive peer relationships; *social*, such as supportive family, socio-economic advantage, and religious and faith affiliations; and *environmental*, such as safe neighbourhoods, connection to pro-social organisations and low community violence (Yates and Masten, 2004).

Individual differences in resilience across the adult life-span are commonly observed. The factors and processes underpinning individual variations in resilience are complex and involve an interplay between a person's competence, their assets and protective resources on the one hand, and the risks, adversity and vulnerabilities they encounter on the other (Yates and Masten, 2004). Competence is the adaptive use of resources within and outside the person, in order to negotiate age-salient developmental challenges and still achieve positive outcomes. Assets and protective factors, as noted above, can take several forms: resources within the community, resources within the person (human capital) and resources within social networks (social capital). Adversity refers to negative experiences or occurrences that have the potential to disrupt adaptive functioning; chronic health conditions are particularly pertinent forms of adversity as people age. Risks refer to the events or conditions that increase the potential for undesired outcomes from adversity but do not necessarily occur for all individuals in a group. In this resilience framework, risks and assets may counterbalance each other and can have cumulative effects and interactions across the life-span (Yates and Masten, 2004). Assets can help people who are in both high- or low-risk situations, whilst protective factors are more salient in helping people in high-risk situations.

Being a multi-faceted concept, resilience has been measured in different ways, with no widely accepted standardised scale currently in use (for a review of resilience measurement scales, see Windle, Bennett and Noyes, 2011). Most scales focus exclusively on personal psychological attributes. The resilience scale developed by Wagnild and Young (1993) focused on the personality characteristic of 'inner strength', defined by the components of equanimity, perseverance, self-reliance, meaningfulness and existential loneliness. The Connor-Davidson Resilience Scale (Connor and Davidson, 2003) includes multiple psychological characteristics of resilient people, such as hardiness, self-efficacy, optimism, action orientation and adaptability to change. The Psychological Resilience Scale (Windle, Markland and Woods, 2008) measures constructs of self-esteem, personal competence and interpersonal control. However, none of these scales include social and environmental factors. There remains a need to develop a multi-dimensional scale of resilience that captures the complexities of the resilience process (Wild, Wiles and Allen, 2013), for unless the multiple domains of resilience are included, the full picture of resilience will not emerge (Kaplan, 2006).

RESILIENCE AND AGEING

There is a growing interest in expanding resilience research across the life course (Kaplan, 1999; Luthar et al., 2000; Richardson, 2002). Research is beginning to examine the resilience of older adults generally (Clark et. al., 2011; Hayslip and Smith, 2012; Lavretsky, 2014; Resnick, Gwyther and Roberto, 2011; Windle, 2011, 2012) and of those living with dementia (Clare et al., 2011; Harris, 2008; Purves et al., 2011). Facing adversities at an older age may be different than at a younger age because of increased vulnerability, loss of important social relationships, loss of meaningful social roles and less effective immune systems (Resnick et al., 2011). Yet, as a group, older adults experience fewer adjustment problems, report less distress and demonstrate better coping in the face of adversity than younger adults with similar problems (Rybarczyk *et al.*, 2012). Theories put forward to explain this group-level phenomenon include: enhanced coping skills from years of facing life-long stressors and illness; stress inoculation from exposure to life-long stressors; more effective emotional regulation; and the development of wisdom and ego transcendence, which provides a more positive and realistic perspective on life (Rybarvzyk *et al.*, 2012). However, currently, relatively little is known about how these personal assets and capabilities contribute to resilience in late life and how they might be maintained (Windle, 2012).

Research has begun to examine factors that might foster resilience as people enter later life. These span a variety of domains and constructs. Socio-cultural factors, ranging from supportive social networks and spiritual support to housing and transportation, have received attention as possible sources of resilience in later life. Sensitivity and attention to ethnic and cultural differences and preferences have also been linked with resilience (see Yee-Melichar, 2011). Positive psychological factors are also being examined, both at the level of certain personality traits, such as optimism, and in relation to psychological coping strategies, such as positive reframing or active problem solving (Lavretsky, 2014; Smith and Hayslip, 2012).

With ageing comes the increased risk of chronic illness. Many older adults face the adversity of living with one or multiple chronic illnesses and/or disabilities but, as a group, they have also been shown to exhibit more resilience in the face of these health challenges than younger adults, again suggesting a role for resilience in relation to coping with long-term health conditions in later life (see Lavretsky, 2014; Rybarczyk *et al.*, 2012). Some studies show how particular positive psychological factors used by people of any age can assist with coping with some chronic diseases. Maintaining optimism helps in recovery from heart disease (e.g. see Scheier *et al.*, 1989), whilst using social support facilitates positive outcomes in a variety of other chronic healthcare conditions, such as cardiovascular disease (Lett *et al.*, 2005), diabetes (White, Richter and Fry, 1992) and cancer (Koopman *et al.*, 1998). Evidence also exists of consistent positive correlations between chronological age, positive coping and psychological adjustment in chronic health problems such as multiple sclerosis and cancer (Bombardier *et al.*, 2010; Cassileth *et al.*, 1984).

RESILIENCE AND DEMENTIA

There is growing evidence that people living with dementia can continue to live meaningful lives with a sense of purpose, maintain reasonable independence and be contributing members of their community (Clare, 2014; Purves *et al.*, 2011; Swaffer, 2014). Since resilience is heavily implicated in adaptation to many other chronic health conditions, it would appear reasonable to predict that living well with dementia will also involve aspects of resilience. However, very few studies to date have examined or demonstrated how using a resilience framework could provide a broader and more comprehensive approach to empowering people with dementia to cope better and live well with the condition. Harris's study (2008) is one of the few that has explicitly applied a resilience framework to dementia, exploring in two in-depth case studies how resilience might contribute to how people live with Alzheimer's disease. The two participants had very different backgrounds, levels of education, life experiences and accomplishments. However, by examining their narratives through a resilience perspective, insight was gained into how both people were managing to live well with Alzheimer's disease and were still actively engaged in living.

The progressive cognitive changes associated with dementia can easily threaten a person's ability to actively maintain positive relationships and, in connection, a positive sense of self. Thus, for a person with dementia to remain or become resilient, more reaching out, more effort, more patience and a willingness to build upon and work with the person's remaining strengths is needed on the part of the person's social network and their community. Structured psycho-social interventions can form part of these endeavours. Purves and colleagues (2011), for example, discuss how narrative-based reminiscence can be used to foster the resilience of a person living with dementia by providing opportunities for positive social interaction and strengthening of relationships, thus increasing the listener's understanding of the unique experiences and strengths of the person and creating the intimacy of a shared experience. However, apart from this, very little is currently known about how the resilience of people living with dementia can be supported at clinical and community levels, and much more research on resilience and dementia is needed (Harris and Keady, 2008).

A STUDY ON RESILIENCE AND DEMENTIA

This section presents a qualitative research study that focused on experiences of resilience in dementia. Resilience was conceptualised in accordance with Windle's (2012) definition described earlier. The research specifically examined whether applying this concept to women living with dementia could uncover resilience-promoting factors (e.g. assets and protective factors) that help such individuals and their families successfully manage and cope. The major research questions driving this study were: 1) 'Is it possible to identify women living with early-stage dementia who display patterns of resilience?' 2) 'What are the common factors across individuals that assist in fostering this resilience process?' Identifying the clinical practice implications of the study's findings in relation to these questions was a key aim.

METHODOLOGY

This research was based on a secondary data analysis of a sub-sample of a larger study (see Harris and Durkin, 2002). The original phenomenological qualitative study focused on gaining a better understanding of the subjective experience of living with early-stage dementia and positive strategies for coping and maintaining a meaningful life.

Research on resilience has followed two major methodological approaches: variable-focused or person-focused. The variable-focused approach examines the relationships and linkages between and among the key components of the theory behind resilience. The person-oriented approach, which often uses case studies, focuses on identifying people who meet the criteria for resilience, particularly in comparison to people with similar levels of risk or adversity who do not exhibit resilience. This approach reflects actual patterns of resilience that occur naturally and emphasises people's lived experiences (Bergman and Magnusson, 1997; Masten, 2001; Masten and Coatsworth, 1998). A person-oriented methodological approach was used in this study of resilience in people with early-stage dementia.

The sample for this study consisted of a sub-sample drawn from the original 2002 study mentioned above. In that study, 20 people living with early stage dementia, aged 54–84 years, were interviewed along with their available caregivers or care-partners. For this study, ten case studies of women were selected, five of whom displayed resilience and five who did not. The presence of resilience was decided by consensus between the person living with dementia, the person's care-partner, the social worker who referred the person to the study and the researcher. Two criteria were used to judge if the process of resilience was occurring: 1) there is now or has been an adversity to overcome; 2) the person is doing all right or 'okay' (Masten and Coatsworth, 1998). In this study, 'okay' related to observable positive outcomes in terms of appropriate healthy functioning and continued engagement in life in spite of dementia (Hayslip and Smith, 2012).

There are many limitations to this kind of qualitative study. The sample was small and certainly does not constitute a representative sample of all women with early-stage dementia. This study also used a cross-sectional approach to the collection of data in order to examine the process of resilience from the perspectives of the participants. However, qualitative research makes no claim to be representative of the population it is examining. The purpose of this methodology is to present a more in-depth, diverse and complex picture of a phenomenon that has been previously reported and to identify possible variables that need to be tested and confirmed in larger representative studies.

FINDINGS

Three major themes relating to the experience of resilience emerged from a comparative qualitative analysis of the ten case studies: 1) *Human Capital* – individual differences that relate to personal assets and capabilities; 2) *Social Capital* – relationship and environmental differences; and 3) *Community Capital* – community resources and opportunity differences.

THEMES OF THE STUDY

1. HUMAN CAPITAL

Three key behaviours (sub-themes) appeared to differentiate people living with dementia who were resilient versus non-resilient: a) acceptance of the diagnosis, b) positive attitude/optimism, and c) active engagement – being a contributing member of society.

Below are some of the narratives that illustrate these points.

a. Acceptance

For those people who were doing 'okay', a key point was that they had been able to accept their diagnosis and move on. That does not mean that they liked it, just that they could accept it. People who were not resilient appeared 'stuck', unable to process and move on from being given a diagnosis of dementia. These differences are illustrated in the following quotes.

- Resilient group:

  > I think that's the point...you have to face it – what's best, what can be done and what can't be done. And take what you have and make something with it. Whatever I can do, I do; if I can't, I don't. Find the best thing you have left and make it bigger.

- Non-resilient group:

  > I feel like at times...I might as well throw in the towel... I'm a has-been.

b. Positive attitude/optimism

Keeping a positive attitude and being 'realistically hopeful' appeared to be another factor that separated the resilient group from the non-resilient group.

- Resilient group:

  > You just have to take the negative and put it behind you, and the positive – try it. I tell myself I am still okay. If something goes wrong, I put it aside and I'll do it later, or maybe I will never get back to it again. But I give myself a choice – maybe I can do this, and if doesn't work, I put it on the cross-off list I can't do any more, so I find something else.

- Non-resilient group:

  > I get very angry at myself because things are not the same. I wonder: 'Where am I going to go and what am I going to do with the rest of my life?' I think of that more than anything.

c. Active engagement /contributing member of society

The resilient women were actively and reciprocally engaged in meaningful activities within their community, whereas members of the non-resilient groups were socially withdrawn.

- Resilient group:

  > I have three friends that we do things together, and they always pick me up. One doesn't cook any more, but I know she likes sweets, so every once in a while I will make bread pudding or rice pudding. That way I can say thank you and give back.

- Non-resilient group:

  > I don't want to embarrass myself. This is a very strong point for me. I just don't work or go out – I used to volunteer at City Hospital. But people talk a lot about things: when someone has something, everyone knows.

Within this theme, the resilient group was characterised by an ability to accept their diagnosis and actively go on living. Their positive attitudes helped them with the daily struggles and doubts they encountered, whilst being actively engaged with meaningful activities helped them cope with and manage dementia positively.

2. SOCIAL CAPITAL

Access to two forms of social resources appeared to differentiate the experiences of resilient and non-resilient participants in this study. Resilient individuals reported having supportive social relationships and/or were experiencing the re-building of connections with family or friends. In addition, they referred to supportive person-centred environments that reinforced acceptance and tolerance and encouraged personal growth.

a. Social relationships

Access to supportive and understanding relationships with family and/or friends clearly impacted the individuals' coping and heavily influenced the experience of resilience.

- Resilient group:

> Well, neither of us were happy that she had this, and I said to myself: 'You are going to have to become a patient person; I know her success depends on it.' And every once in a while, she will surprise me with a solution to a problem that was right in front of me. Sometimes I begin to put too little importance on her comments and I realise how wrong I am for devaluing her opinion.
>
> *(Friend)*

- Non-resilient group:

> This is like going into a bad dream that starts out as a nightmare. I feel robbed of life, freedom and personhood.
>
> *(Carer)*

b.   *Supportive person-centred environment*

People's narratives illustrated the importance of a supportive person-centred environment that was accepting of a person for who they were, and that supported their agency and involvement.

- Resilient group:

> The hardest part for me is to try to help her keep her independence... She is in on all relevant decisions; we talk things out. I think that type of thing is important for her to be involved. She still has an opinion; just because she doesn't remember doesn't mean she doesn't have an opinion about things.
>
> *(Carer)*

- Non-resilient group:

> Someone has to take command. Someone has to be in charge... There is no relationship to speak of; no repartee; there's no intelligent conversation; and I like being around smart people. She has become plain vanilla.
>
> *(Carer)*

These narratives clearly indicate that having supportive family and friends and a supportive accepting environment – a 'home' in the true sense of the word – were resilience-promoting factors that helped these participants to live with dementia.

3. COMMUNITY CAPITAL

The final theme that differentiated resilient from non-resilient individuals encompassed their connections with community resources and healthcare professionals. Resilient people were connected and took advantage of supportive opportunities and resources available to them. They were integrated into a community, involved with the Alzheimer's Association, taking part in physical exercise programmes, doing volunteer work or involved in church/temple activities and connecting with neighbours. The non-resilient individuals experienced isolation, had limited connections to healthcare providers and used limited support resources available to them.

- Resilient group:

    When I first went to see my doctor, I told him I thought I had some signs of Alzheimer's, and at first he told me, 'I don't think you are right', but after some tests he told me it was Alzheimer's and gave me his phone number to call him any time with any questions I had. He told me to focus on what I can do, not what I can't do.

- Non-resilient group:

    The Memory Centre is such a depressing place to go. I feel once my doctor gave me the diagnosis, he gave up on me.

To summarise, the study's findings suggest certain types of assets and protective factors are involved in the experience of resilience in early-stage dementia. These include particular aspects of human capital – acceptance of the diagnosis, keeping a positive/optimistic outlook and being actively engaged in community-based activities that are meaningful. In addition, keeping, or reconnecting with, friends and family and living in an environment that is accepting, non-judgemental and sensitive to the person's capabilities also appear to be resilience-promoting. In other words, having strong social capital is likely to help a person with dementia get through difficult challenges in life, perhaps because this fosters and maintains the assets and competence involved in having strong human capital. Finally, having a positive relationship with healthcare providers and using available community resources (community capital) could be important in managing and coping with dementia.

PRACTICE IMPLICATIONS

What does applying a resilience framework mean for living well with dementia? How do we apply these findings to clinical practice? As Cacioppo, Reis and Zatura (2011) state, the biggest challenges are being able to identify the individual, social and group structures that promote resilience and provide the basis for the development of interventions. The study described earlier indicates how certain behaviours, which it might be possible for people living with dementia to learn or re-learn, could be actively fostered by clinicians in order to maintain resilience and living well with dementia (see Table 6.1).

Table 6.1: Potential interventions for fostering resilience in people living with dementia

RESILIENCE-PROMOTING FACTORS	POTENTIAL INTERVENTIONS
Acceptance	Obtain accurate information about dementia and discuss with the person.
	Assure the person they are not to blame for the disease and work to dispel myths surrounding dementia.
	Provide opportunities in a safe environment for the expression of feelings including frustration, anger, guilt, blame, hopelessness and humiliation.
	Help the person with dementia move towards acknowledgement of the dementia diagnosis through post-diagnostic counselling.
	Discuss how diagnosis has affected family and other relationships.
	Work with people to understand that they can be a partner in decision making.
	Encourage joining support groups online or in person.
Optimism/hope	Help the person with dementia to identify life-long strengths and new strengths – look for examples of resiliency and adaptation.
	Make a list of the person's accomplishments.
	Help the person with dementia to explore, discuss and identify previous positive coping strategies.

Active engagement	Reframe loss as an opportunity, not a failure.
	Assist in identifying life-long skills, interests and passions.
	Discuss how these can be adapted to continue to be part of the person's life.
	Address ways family members and friends can assist in these endeavours (e.g. transportation, joining in the activity if necessary).
Supportive social relationships	Encourage people with dementia and family members to acknowledge the dementia to close friends.
	Encourage people living with dementia to discuss positive ways in which family members or friends can assist them in maintaining reasonable independence and involvement in life.
	Encourage family members to listen.
Supportive person-centred environment	Discuss with the family the need to treat people living with dementia as capable and as partners in their future planning process.
	Provide opportunities for people and families to address feelings of loss of social roles.
	Identify actions that can diminish people's feelings of self-worth.
	Collaborate with people living with dementia and their families in advocating for making communities that are more dementia-friendly.
Connection to community resources and healthcare professionals	Encourage and follow up on referral to support groups (online or in person).
	Make referrals to dementia-friendly healthcare professionals and institutions, and follow up.
	Have the person rehearse asking questions about health or social concerns to prepare them for their appointments.
	Encourage involvement in other community resources.

CONCLUSIONS

The concept of resilience helps to highlight key behaviours and resources (resilience-promoting factors) that people living with dementia might possibly (re)learn and that clinicians and family members might be able to foster in order to promote living well. Learned behaviours that are facilitated by supportive social resources could constitute important competences and assets that enable people to withstand adversity in dementia and use positive coping strategies that maintain well-being. Applying a resilience framework in dementia care and support services could provide opportunities for people living with dementia to live a life of meaning, not despite the disease, but with the disease. Our role as clinicians, researchers, family members, friends and, most importantly, citizens, is to recognise the strengths, assets and resources of people living with dementia and develop practices, environments and communities that are dementia-friendly and oriented towards building and preserving resilience. For we should want all people living with dementia to believe, as one resilient woman stated, 'I am not afraid if I don't remember or if something doesn't work out. I know we'll try something else. So it is not a threat to me. And I feel okay.'

REFERENCES

Allen, R.S., Haley, P.P., Harris, G.M., Fowler, S.N. and Pruthi, R. (2011) 'Resilience, Definitions, Ambiguities, and Applications.' In B. Resnick, L.P. Gwyther, and K.A. Roberto (eds) *Resilience in Aging: Concepts, Research and Outcomes*. New York, NY: Springer.

Baltes, P.B. and Baltes, M.M. (1990) *Successful Ageing: Perspectives from Behavioural Science*. Cambridge: Cambridge University Press.

Bergman, L.R. and Magnusson, D. (1997) 'A person-oriented approach in research on developmental psychopathology.' *Development and Psychopathology 9*, 291–319.

Bombardier, C.H., Ehde, D.M., Stoelb, B. and Molton, I.R. (2010) 'The relationship of age related factors to psychological functioning among people with disabilities.' *Physical Medicine and Rehabilitation Clinics of North America 21*(2), 281–297.

Cacioppo, J.T., Reis, H.T. and Zautra, A.J. (2011) 'Social resilience: The value of social fitness with an application to the military.' *The American Psychologist 66*(1), 43–51.

Cassileth, B.R., Lusk, E.J., Strouse, T.B., Miller, D.S. *et al.* (1984) 'Psychosocial status in chronic illness: A comparative analysis of six diagnostic groups.' *The New England Journal of Medicine 311*(8), 506–511.

Cicchetti, D., Rappaport, J., Sandler, L. and Weissberg, R.P. (eds) (2000) *The Promotion of Wellness in Children and Adolescents*. Washington, DC: Child Welfare League of America.

Clare, L., Kinsella, G.L., Logsdon, R., Whitlatch, C. and Zarit, S. (2011) 'Building Resilience in Mild Cognitive Impairment and Early-stage Dementia: Innovative Approaches to Intervention and Outcome Evaluations.' In B. Resnick, L.P. Gwyther and K.A. Roberto (eds) *Resilience in Aging: Concepts, Research and Outcomes*. New York, NY: Springer.

Clare, L. , Nelis, S. M., Quinn, C., Martyr, A., *et al.* (2014) 'Improving the experience of dementia and enhancing active life – living well with dementia: Study protocol for the ideal study.' *Health and Quality Life Outcomes 12*(1), 164–179.

Clark, P., Burbank, M., Greene, G., Owens, N. and Riebe, D. (2011) 'What Do We Know About Resilience in Older Adults? An Exploration of Some Facts, Factors, and Facets.' In B. Resnick, L.P. Gwyther and K. Roberto. (eds) *Resilience in Aging: Concepts, Research and Outcomes*. New York, NY: Springer.

Connor, K.M. and Davidson J.R.T. (2003) 'The development of a new resilience scale: The Connor–Davidson Resilience Scale (CD-RISC).'*Depression and Anxiety 18*, 76–82.

Hardy, S.E., Concato, J. and Gill, T.M. (2002) 'Stressful life events among community-living older people.' *Journal of General Internal Medicine 17*, 841–847.

Harris, P.B. (2008) 'Another wrinkle in the debate about successful ageing: The undervalued concept of resilience and the lived experience of dementia.' *International Journal of Ageing and Human Development 67*(1), 43–61.

Harris, P.B. and Durkin, C. (2002) 'Building Resilience Through Coping and Adapting.' In P.B. Harris (ed.) *The Person With Alzheimer's Disease: Pathways to Understanding the Experience*. Baltimore, MD: John Hopkins University Press.

Harris, P.B. and Keady, J. (2008) 'Wisdom, resilience and successful ageing: Changing public discourses on living with dementia.' *Dementia 7*(1), 5–8.

Hayslip, B. and Smith, G. (2012) 'Resilience in Adulthood and Later Life: What Does It Mean and Where Are We Headed?' In B. Hayslip, and G. Smith (eds) *Annual Review of Gerontology and Geriatrics: Emerging Perspectives on Resilience and Adulthood and Later Life*. New York: Springer.

Holstein, M.B. and Minkler, M. (2003) 'Self, society, and the "new gerontology."' *The Gerontologist 43*(6), 787–796.

Kahana, E. and Kahana, B. (1996) 'Conceptual and Empirical Advances in Understanding Ageing Well Through Protective Adaptation.' In V. Bengtson (ed.) *Adulthood and Ageing: Research on Continuities and Discontinuities*. New York, NY: Springer Publishing.

Kahana, E. and Kahana, B. (2003) 'Contextualising Successful Ageing: New Directions in an Age-Old Search.' In Richard Settersten Jr. (ed.) *Invitation to the Life Course: Toward New Understanding of Late Life*. Amityville, NY: Bayword Publishing.

Kaplan, H.B. (1999) 'Toward an Understanding of Resilience: A Critical Review of Definitions and Models.' In M. Glanz and J.L. Johnson (eds) *Resilience and Development: Positive Life Adaptations*. New York, NY: Plenum.

Kaplan. H.B. (2006) 'Understanding the Concept of Resilience.' In S. Goldstein and R.B. Brooks (eds) *Handbook of Resilience in Children*. New York, NY: Springer.

Katz, S. and Calasanti, T. (2015) 'Critical perspectives on successful ageing: Does it "appeal more than it illuminates"?' *The Gerontologist 55*(1), 26–33.

Koopman, C., Hermanson, K., Diamond, S., Angell, K. and Spiegel, D. (1998) 'Social support, life stress, pain and emotional adjustment to advanced breast cancer.' *Psycho-oncology* 7(2), 101–111.

Lavretsky, H. (2014) *Resilience and Ageing Research and Practice*. Baltimore, MD: Johns Hopkins University Press.

Lett, H.S., Blumenthal, J.A., Babyak, M.A., Strauman, T.J., Robins, C. and Sherwood, A. (2005) 'Social support and coronary heart disease: Epidemiological evidence and implications for treatment.' *Psychosomatic Medicine* 67(6), 869–878.

Luthar, S.S. (1999) 'Measurement Issues in the Empirical Study of Resilience: An Overview.' In M. Glanz and J.L. Johnson (eds) *Resilience and Development: Positive Life Adaptations*. New York, NY: Plenum.

Luthar, S., Cicchetti, D. and Becker, B. (2000) 'The construct of resilience: A critical evaluation and guidelines for future work.' *Child Development* 71(3), 543–562.

Luthar, S.S. and Zelazo, L.B. (2003) 'Research on Resilience.' In Suniya S. Luthar (ed.) *Reliance and Vulnerability: Adaptation in the Context of Childhood Adversity*. New York, NY: Cambridge University Press.

Martinson, M. and Berridge, C. (2015) 'Successful ageing and its discontents: A systematic review of the social gerontology literature.' *The Gerontologist* 55(1), 58–69.

Masten, A.S. (2001) 'Ordinary magic: Resilience processes in development.' *American Psychologist* 56(3), 227–238.

Masten, A.S. and Coatsworth, J.D. (1998) 'The development of competence in favourable and unfavourable environments: Lessons from successful children.' *American Psychologist* 53, 205–222.

Purves, B., Savundranayagam, M.Y., Kelson, E., Astell, A. and Phinney, A. (2011) 'Fostering Resilience in Dementia through Narratives: Contributions of Multimedia Technology.' In B. Resnick, L.P. Gwyther and K.A. Roberto (eds) *Resilience in Aging: Concepts, Research and Outcomes*. New York, NY: Springer.

Resnick, B., Gwyther, L.P. and Roberto, K.A. (eds) (2011) *Resilience in Aging: Concepts, Research and Outcomes*. New York, NY: Springer.

Richardson, G.E. (2002) 'The metatheory of resilience and resiliency.' *Journal of Clinical Psychology* 58, 307–321.

Rowe, J.W. and Kahn, R.I. (1997) 'Successful ageing.' *The Gerontologist* 37, 433–480.

Rowe, J.W. and Kahn, R.I. (1998) *Successful Ageing: The MacArthur Foundation Study*. New York, NY: Pantheon.

Rybarczyk, B., Emery, E.E., Guequierre, L.L., Shamaskin, A. and Behel, J. (2012) 'The Role of Resilience in Chronic Illness and Disability in Older Adults.' In B. Hayslip and G.C. Smith (eds) *Annual Review of Gerontology and Geriatrics: Emerging Perspectives on Resilience in Later Life (vol. 32)*.New York, NY: Springer Publishing.

Scheier, M.F., Matthews, K.A., Owens, J.F., Magovern, G.J. *et al.* (1989) 'Dispositional optimism and recovery from coronary artery bypass surgery: The beneficial effects on physical and psychological well-being.' *Journal of Personality and Social Psychology* 57(6), 1024–1040.

Smith, G.C. and Hayslip, B. (2012) 'Resilience in Adulthood and Later Life.' In B. Hayslip and G.C. Smith (eds) *Annual Review of Gerontology and Geriatrics: Emerging Perspectives on Resilience in Later Life (vol. 32)*.New York, NY: Springer.

Sterin, G.J. (2002) 'Essay on a word: A lived experience of Alzheimer's disease.' *Dementia 1*(1), 7–10.

Swaffer, K. (2014) 'Stigma, language, dementia friendly.' *Dementia 13*(6), 709–716.

Swaffer, K. (2015) 'Dementia and Prescribed DisengagementTM.' *Dementia 14*(1), 3–6.

Vaillant, G.E. (2004) 'Positive Ageing.' In A. Linley and S. Joseph (eds) *Positive Psychology in Practice*. New York, NY: John Wiley & Sons, Inc.

Wagnild, G.M. and Young, H.M. (1993) 'Development and psychometric evaluation of the resilience scale.' *Journal of Nursing Measurement 1*(2), 165–178.

White, N.E., Richter, J.M. and Fry, C. (1992) 'Coping, social support, and adaptation to chronic illness.' *Western Journal of Nursing Research 14*(2), 211–224.

Wild, K., Wiles, J.L. and Allen, R.E.S. (2013) 'Resilience: Thoughts on the value of the concept for critical gerontology.' *Ageing and Society 33*(1), 137–158.

Wiles, J.L., Wild, K., Kerse, N. and Allen, R.E.S. (2012) 'Resilience from the point of view of older people: There is still life beyond the funny bone.' *Social Science and Medicine 74*(3), 416–424.

Windle, G. (2011) 'What is resilience? A review and concept analysis.' *Reviews in Clinical Gerontology 21*, 152–169.

Windle, G. (2012) 'The contribution of resilience to healthy ageing.' *Perspectives in Public Health 132*(4), 159–160.

Windle, G., Bennett, K.M. and Noyes, J. (2011) 'A methodological review of resilience measurement scales.' *Health and Quality Outcomes 9*(8), 1–18.

Windle, G., Markland, D.A. and Woods, R.T. (2008) 'Examination of a theoretical model of psychological resilience in older age.' *Ageing and Mental Health 12*(3), 285–292.

Yates, T.M. and Masten, A.S. (2004) 'Fostering the Future: Resilience Theory and Practice of Positive Psychology.' In P.A. Linley and S. Joseph (eds) *Positive Psychology in Practice*. New York, NY: John Wiley & Sons, Inc.

Yee-Melichar, D. (2011) 'Resilience in ageing: Cultural and Ethnic Perspectives.' In B. Resnick, L.P. Gwyther and K.A. Roberto (eds) *Resilience in Aging: Concepts, Research and Outcomes*. New York, NY: Springer.

Chapter 7

GROWTH

Kirsty Patterson and Emma Wolverson

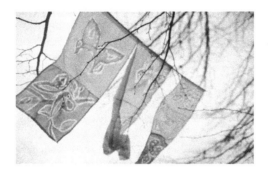

Most, if not all, of us will be able to look back on a time when we knew less, cared too much – or perhaps even too little. In large or small ways, we are able to look at ourselves now and say, 'I am wiser/stronger/better than before.' Some of these changes may have transpired almost without us noticing, whilst others may have been set in motion deliberately as we explored new ways to better ourselves. Throughout life, the drive to develop and grow as people helps us to overcome our fears, achieve our goals, develop stronger relationships and push past personal boundaries and plateaus. In short, through growing personally we get to know and understand ourselves better and connect more deeply with the world around us.

What happens, then, when we reach later life? Some societal narratives portray old age as a time of stagnation or even decline, but other contrasting narratives associate advancing age with increasing wisdom and self-acceptance. What happens too, when our goals and progress are interrupted by significant events, such as a serious illness?

Although it is recognised that illness can cause considerable distress, we are all likely to have heard stories in which an individual has harnessed their illness as a catalyst to alter their whole outlook on life and foster new and meaningful goals. From these questions arises another: can people gain wisdom, grow and experience a new outlook on life whilst living with dementia?

These are the questions we explore throughout this chapter. We begin by offering a definition of what it means to 'grow', followed by an introduction to two dominant perspectives on growth within the literature: that of growth as a natural part of life-span development and that of growth as a response to adversity. We use these perspectives to consider how growth may be related to the experiences of older people and to the experiences of people living with illness. We draw upon these two perspectives and the current empirical literature to consider the potential for growth in the context of dementia.

DEFINING GROWTH

Growth can be defined as a positive change in our psychological functioning (Tedeschi and Calhoun, 2004), in which we develop beyond a previous version of ourselves. Through growth we gain something new and positive in relation to our ability to fit or function in our environment or in our level of awareness about ourselves and the life we lead (Zoellner and Maercker, 2006). However, it is difficult to put too fine a definition around such a broad concept and around one that is such a subjective and individual experience.

Growth overlaps with a number of related concepts, such as thriving, flourishing and optimal functioning. Thriving has been defined as a process of reaching a higher level of psychological functioning (Carver, 1998). Similarly, flourishing and optimal functioning have been ascribed to a higher range of human functioning, 'one that connotes goodness, generativity, *growth*, and resilience' (Fredrickson and Losada, 2005, p.678). What unites these concepts is a shared understanding that the absence of negative psychological states is not always sufficient for psychological well-being (Keyes, 2002). To flourish, thrive or grow is to do more than to avoid languishing (Fredrickson and Losada, 2005) or stagnation – it implies moving beyond a comfortable baseline, venturing into new possibilities of life and meaning. However, what the concept of growth adds is the potential for growth to exist alongside negative psychological states or even be stimulated by them (Tedeschi and Calhoun, 2004) – an issue discussed later.

According to Ryff and Keyes (1995), growth is one of six key features of psychological well-being – of equal importance to positive relationships, self-acceptance, autonomy, environmental mastery and purpose in life. Such an understanding of psychological well-being takes us beyond the notion that well-being is created simply by feelings of happiness. This model instead highlights the importance of eudemonic well-being, which involves having a sense of meaning and purpose in life (Ryff and Singer, 2008), realising and actualising one's true potential and living according to one's true self and values (Deci and Ryan, 2008). Thus, whilst growth can lead us to heightened well-being, each person's journey of self-discovery and development will be unique.

GROWTH THROUGH THE LIFE-SPAN

Humanistic and life-span development psychological theories portray growth as a life-long, natural and universal process. We possess strong needs to develop our cognitive abilities, to experience new and beautiful sights, to actualise our full potential and to transcend previous definitions of ourselves (Maslow, 1954). We find value in experiences that foster our long-term development (Rogers, 1959). As Fromm (1955, p.25) said, 'The whole life of the individual is nothing but the process of giving birth to himself; indeed, we should be fully born when we die.' According to Organismic Valuing Process (OVP) theory, we all have the capacity to know what values will satisfy and enhance us along our life path and can take corrective action where necessary if our life has deviated from this path (Rogers, 1951). In Erikson's (1963) model of psycho-social development, individuals are understood to progress through a series of transitional stages throughout their life-span. Each stage presents a different challenge to personal and social development and represents a crossroad, a point from which the individual can either regress or progress (Erikson, 1963). If the individual is able to resolve the necessary psychological tasks of a stage, they are enabled to move forwards – developing their sense of self and fostering strengths or virtues that will assist them with future challenges.

Although growth is a natural and life-long process, do all individuals grow to the same degree? And what outcomes might we expect in people who have experienced growth? Maslow's (1954, 1969) hierarchy of motivation suggests that an individual's more basic physical and psychological needs must be met before they can be motivated to fulfil their potential – suggesting therefore that those whose basic needs are not always met may have fewer opportunities to pursue growth and self-development. Similarly, both the OVP theory (Rogers, 1951) and Erikson's (1963) life-span model recognise that, whilst the capacity for growth throughout the life-span may be innate, the extent to which this can occur may be influenced by various internal and external factors impacting upon the individual, including the conditions within their social environment. This is important to consider, given the malignant social contexts surrounding people with dementia (Kitwood, 1990) and the ongoing struggle for overstretched, underfunded residential care facilities to do more than meet people's basic physical needs.

Some theorists have presented us with a picture of what an individual may grow into, given the right environmental conditions. Rogers (1959) suggests that when an individual becomes 'fully functioning', they are able to understand and accept themselves as they are, to live in the moment, find meaning in their lives, and find value in compassionate relationships as well as the authenticity of self and others. However, Rogers adds that to be fully functioning is also to be in a process of continual change and progression. Similarly, Maslow (1954) suggests that striving to self-actualise – in other words, to reach one's full potential – can be best thought of as a process of *becoming* oneself. If the process of growth is never complete, then capturing its outcomes becomes very difficult.

Furthermore, growth may not be restricted to changes within an individual's sense of self. The concept of transcendence, or self-transcendence, has been described as a process of developing beyond one's individual identity and needs, towards an identity that is increasingly linked to others and the wider universe (Reed, 1991). Transcendence has been placed at the top of Maslow's (1969) updated hierarchy of motivation; whilst the self-actualising individual reaches towards their own potential, the self-transcending individual goes one step further, developing 'beyond themselves' and identifying with something greater (Koltko-Rivera, 2006). It seems therefore that the process of growth may be as long and as broad as could be imagined.

GROWTH IN OLDER PEOPLE

If growth is a life-long process, then it is conceivable that the heights of personal growth are reached in our older years, after a life-time spent developing our sense of self and ways of relating. As Jung (1970, p.787) suggests:

> A human being would certainly not grow to be seventy or eighty years old if this longevity had no meaning for the species. The afternoon of human life must also have a significance of its own and cannot be merely a pitfall to life's morning.

An aspect of human development that is often associated with the 'afternoon' of the life-span is the gaining of wisdom. Psychology lacks a single definition of wisdom (see Chapter 9 for more discussion of the concept). It has been described as a process of cognitive development (whereby people develop a rich factual and procedural knowledge) and life-span contextualism (i.e. knowledge about the relative unpredictability of life and ways to manage) (Baltes and Staudinger, 2000). Others have regarded wisdom as an advanced stage of personality development, whereby a person, over the course of their life-span, develops expertise in the conduct and meaning of life (Erikson, 1963).

The development of wisdom was initially the end-point of Erikson's (1963) theory of life-span development (at age 65+). However, Erikson and Erikson (1997) later added a final (ninth) stage of development – that of gerotranscendence. The notion of gerotranscendence was first put forward by Tornstam (1989) and is consistent with the idea that growth is a life-long process that peaks in old age. Tornstam suggests that as people grow older, they often experience an important shift in perspective, leading them to re-define themselves and their relationships, and develop new ways of being in the world, in turn fostering a heightened sense of life satisfaction. Tornstam (2011) describes three key domains within which people can develop:

1. Within the domain of 'the self', people may come to consider the different parts of themselves, uncovering both good and bad, but developing an acceptance of themselves and the life

that has been lived. They may reduce their focus upon their own needs to increasingly focus upon the needs of others.

2. In the 'relational' domain, people may grow to focus more selectively upon those relationships that are most important to them and may feel more of a need for solitude. They can become more tolerant and open-minded, less materialistic and less concerned with abiding by social conventions and upholding social roles.

3. Within the 'cosmic domain', people may develop a different perspective on time, life and death as they age. They feel more connected to others around them and to the generations preceding and succeeding them, whilst finding greater joy in daily experiences.

Whilst some research findings indicate that older people experience a sense of growth in these domains (e.g. Tornstam, 2005; Wadensten, 2005), studies also highlight significant variations in growth across different domains and between individuals, presumably based on varying life experiences. For example, older people have expressed varying levels of agreement with different statements about growth (Tornstam, 2005) on the Gerotranscendence Scale (Braam *et al.*, 2006; Tornstam, 1999; Tornstam, 2011). Patterns of growth have also been found to differ across genders and have been associated to varying degrees with other factors, such as relationship status and the presence of adverse events (Tornstam, 2005). For example, cosmic transcendence has been found to be positively associated with negative life events in later life; and, in fact, transcendence in this domain has been found to *decrease* over time where no negative life events are experienced (Read *et al.*, 2014). Such findings indicate that there may be individual differences in trajectories of personal growth in later life and that growth across the life-span might be additionally stimulated following adversity. If the presence of dementia or the process of its diagnosis is experienced as a negative life event, it is possible that cosmic growth is particularly relevant to older people living with dementia. We shall therefore now consider the theoretical and empirical literature around growth stimulated by adversity.

GROWTH IN RESPONSE TO ADVERSITY

We have considered the notion that we may gradually grow and develop throughout our lives, as we negotiate life's transitions and steer ourselves towards pathways of fulfilment. But what happens when sudden or unexpected life events suddenly throw us off our normal trajectory? People can experience a range of distressing psychological problems and negative outcomes following traumatic or adverse circumstances. However, a body of literature has also explored the notion that people, rather than remaining unchanged by trauma, can in fact change in positive ways *because* of it (Tedeschi and Calhoun, 2004). That particular kinds of strength might emerge from traumatic circumstances has been explored in both literary fiction as well as psychology. In the novel *A Farewell to Arms*, for example, Ernest Hemingway writes that 'The world breaks everyone, and afterward, some are strong at the broken places' (2012/1929, p.216). Such post-traumatic growth, or PTG, is thought to lie beyond resilience since, as Hemingway implies, the individual surpasses, rather than returns to, previous levels of functioning (Carver, 1998). This is not to suggest that PTG is a *better* outcome than resilience or coping. Simply, it offers another valid and valuable human response to adversity, where 'particular heights of human experience' can be reached by 'those who have run the gauntlet' (Ryff and Singer, 2003, p.16).

For some, the experience of growth following adversity has been understood as a process of cognitive appraisal, used to cope with and make meaning out of difficult life events (Davis, Nolen-Hoeksema and Larson, 1998; Filipp, 1999; Park and Folkman, 1997; Taylor, 1983) – for example, by finding benefits within the event (Davis *et al.*, 1998) or enhancing one's perceived ability to cope with future difficulties (Taylor, 1983). It has been claimed that perceptions of growth are 'illusory' coping mechanisms (Zoellner and Maercker, 2006), used to adjust to difficult experiences rather than to develop oneself positively – if these appraisals do not translate into objective changes in lifestyle (Hobfoll *et al.*, 2007). Although a number of quantitative, self-report questionnaires have been developed to measure levels of PTG (for a review, see Joseph and Linley, 2008), these rely upon accurate retrospective accounts of changes in functioning, and some have suggested that people are biased towards perceiving that they have changed positively over time (McFarland and Alvaro, 2000).

Still, a number of theorists maintain that growth *can* be stimulated specifically by traumatic events, and that this growth can transcend the cognitive level – transforming the individual in positive and meaningful ways. It is suggested that deliberate cognitive effort is needed (often aided by self-disclosure and social support) to process events that have initially shattered a person's assumptions about the world and impaired their psychological functioning, and that this processing is thought to facilitate the person in restructuring and developing their life narrative; ultimately enabling them to grow beyond previous levels of functioning (Joseph and Linley, 2005; Tedeschi and Calhoun, 2004). The transformations that may be involved in PTG have been described (Joseph and Linley, 2005) in relation to:

- growth of the self (e.g. feeling that one has become stronger or wiser as a person, or becoming more accepting of one's weaknesses and limitations)

- interpersonal growth (e.g. an enhanced appreciation of one's relationships, or a heightened sense of compassion towards others)

- existential growth (e.g. the re-evaluation of one's priorities or an increased appreciation of life, created within a context of realising one's mortality).

Given these varied perspectives on PTG, how do we know that growth is 'authentic' (i.e. distinct from adjustment) in response to difficult life events? Perhaps it is possible that growth following adversity may at times reflect a cognitive coping strategy (which may be very helpful to people in its own right), and may at other times reflect a more transformative experience. It is also possible that both forms of growth may occur within the same individual at different points in time. This notion is consistent with the finding that growth following adversity is, in the short term, most strongly associated with reduced negative mental health, but in the longer term is most strongly associated with positive psychological health (Helgeson, Reynolds and Tomich, 2006; Sawyer, Ayers and Field, 2010). This may support the idea that, initially, people's efforts are directed towards emotional management (Tedeschi and Calhoun, 2004) and perceptions of growth represent a coping strategy based on benefit finding. Over time, however, some individuals may focus their efforts upon finding meaning and creating positive changes.

GROWTH THROUGH ILLNESS

A growing body of research attests to the potential for growth through the experience of illness, most commonly focusing upon cancer-related illnesses. In a review by Koutrouli, Anagnostopoulos and Potamianos (2012), for example, all 12 of the included studies found that the majority of their participants perceived themselves to have experienced PTG through living with breast cancer. In one of these studies by Weiss (2002), 98 per cent of participants with breast cancer agreed with statements on the Posttraumatic Growth Inventory (Tedeschi and Calhoun, 1996), such as 'I discovered that I'm stronger than I thought I was.' One issue with the research in this area is that studies have not typically included a control group and so it is difficult to know if perceived growth was stimulated by illness specifically, or if it would have occurred naturally over time through developmental processes (Eve and Kangas, 2015; Koutrouli *et al.*, 2012).

Qualitative research has enabled further insight into the subjective experience of growth through illness, mainly focused again upon cancer-related illnesses. A meta-synthesis conducted by Hefferon, Grealy and Mutrie (2009) indicated that participants' experiences of growth broadly map onto the three areas of growth highlighted in models of PTG: development of the self, existential re-evaluation, and the prioritisation of relationships (the latter of which was part of a larger theme around the re-appraisal of life and one's priorities). In addition, a fourth area of growth was identified, which was suggested to be potentially unique to PTG following physical illness: an increased awareness and sense of connection to the physical self, with subsequent positive changes in health behaviours.

Together, this literature highlights how illness may act as a catalyst to growth and that, as a result of their illness experience, people perceive themselves to have changed in positive and meaningful ways. Might this be the case too for people living with dementia? Before exploring this possibility in full, it is worth considering aspects of dementia that may differ from physical health conditions previously linked to PTG and, therefore, how growth might be experienced and expressed in dementia. The following might be some points to consider:

- *Social acceptability and stigma* – Physical illnesses such as cancer remain more socially accepted than dementia, which can still be met with considerable stigma (e.g. O'Sullivan, Hocking and Spence, 2014). PTG has been found to be positively associated with seeking social (Koutrouli *et al.*, 2012) and emotional support from others (Barskova and Oesterreich, 2009) and having contact with another individual who has experienced growth (Koutrouli *et al.*, 2012), as supportive others may assist the individual to develop a narrative about their experiences and construct new meaning from it (Tedeschi and Calhoun, 2004). It is worth considering the extent to which people living with dementia are supported to develop narratives pertaining to growth in the context of their condition.

- *Differences associated with age* – There is evidence to suggest that higher levels of PTG following illness are found in younger adults compared to older adults (e.g. Barskova and Oesterreich, 2009), which could suggest that PTG processes are less applicable to older people living with dementia. This may be due to a ceiling effect, whereby older people, who have been growing and maturing throughout life, have less room to grow further in the context of illness (Eve and Kangas, 2015; Tedeschi and Calhoun, 2004). Alternatively, any apparent impact of age may depend upon how we choose to define and measure growth. For example, Barskova and Oesterreich (2009) identified no significant effect of age when measures of growth focused upon changes in family relationships, acceptance and views about the world (e.g. Benefit Finding Scale – Tomich and Helgeson, 2004) – domains of growth that may be more relevant to older people compared to other measures.

- *Issues of severity, chronicity and prognosis* – The literature on growth through illness has largely focused on the experiences of survivors or people with early stage physical illnesses (Tang *et al.*, 2015). This questions its applicability to those living with more chronic illnesses or those facing a poor prognosis. There is some evidence that illnesses of moderate severity are most conducive to growth since these are sufficiently severe to create a shattering and rebuilding of assumptions, but not so severe as to overwhelm the individual's resources and ability to find meaning and engender change (Barskova and Osterreich, 2009). However, evidence of growth has been found in individuals with advanced and terminal cases of illness (Montoya-Juarez *et al.*, 2013; Mystakidou *et al.*, 2008; Tang *et al.*, 2015).

Furthermore, there is evidence of growth in people living with long-term, chronic and progressive conditions, including long-term disabilities (e.g. Kampman *et al.*, 2015), HIV/AIDS (e.g. Sawyer *et al.*, 2010), multiple sclerosis (Pakenham, 2007) and stroke (Gillen, 2005). The findings of one meta-synthesis indicate that growth in chronic illness may follow an oscillating, rather than strictly linear, pattern. Paterson (2001) suggests that people living with chronic illness will at times focus upon the loss and suffering it induces, but at other times they may find a way to frame their illness as a meaningful opportunity to create positive changes in life. A similarly oscillating pattern of adjustment has been described within the lived experience literature in dementia (Robinson, Clare and Evans, 2005). It is therefore possible that dementia may at times be experienced as a burden but at other times experienced as a catalyst for change by the same individual.

• *The impact of cognitive ability* – PTG has been understood as a process of cognitive appraisal (Davis *et al.*, 1998; Filipp, 1999; Park and Folkman, 1997; Taylor, 1983), or a transformative experience that emerges following the deliberate cognitive processing of difficult events (Joseph and Linley, 2005; Tedeschi and Calhoun, 2004). This raises questions as to whether the cognitive impairments associated with dementia would interfere with the processing necessary for PTG.

With these similarities and differences in mind, we now move on to consider the current evidence base regarding the potential for growth amongst people living with dementia.

GROWTH AND DEMENTIA – IS IT POSSIBLE?

Since writing my first book, and grappling with the fear of ceasing to be, I have worked through what it means to be 'me', and have been able to answer the question it posed. I realise what it is that I am losing, and what will always remain. I now know that in this journey towards my true self, with dementia stripping away the layers of cognition and emotion, I'm becoming who I really am.

Christine Bryden, Dancing with Dementia: My Story of Living Positively with Dementia *(2005, p.162)*

When people talk about older people with dementia, they are intuitively more likely to use terms such as *slowing, stopping, losing, declining, deteriorating* and *regressing*, rather than terms such as *growing, developing* and *transcending*. But are we right to exclude older people with dementia from conversations about growth?

Research exploring the subjective experience of growth in caregivers of people living with dementia (e.g. Peacock *et al.*, 2010) has identified that whilst the caregiving experience can generate strains, it can also generate positive gains relating to personal development, new opportunities and connectedness to others, including the person for whom they provide care (see Chapter 11).

What about the other side of the dyad? If dementia can provide caregivers with opportunities to learn, discover, re-evaluate and find meaning within their experiences, might this not also be the case for people navigating the condition itself? A small body of literature has begun to shed some light on these questions. Kitwood (1995, p.135) noted:

> In the course of my own involvement with those who have dementia, now spanning almost ten years, I have come across several striking instances of positive long-term change. There are even two persons alive today, with severe dementia…who appear now to be in a higher state of overall well-being than they were at the time when I first knew them.

Other healthcare professionals surveyed by Kitwood were able to provide retrospective accounts of 49 other persons with dementia who had experienced a range of positive changes – most commonly – increased assertiveness, increased warmth and affection, higher levels of trust, greater acceptance of limitations, heightened spontaneity, as well as transcending depression and overcoming shame. Kitwood (1995) concluded that some of these changes likely marked a return to personality traits that had been temporarily disrupted by the onset of dementia but, in other cases, reflected the development of new ways of living and being; a kind of 'personal growth' (Kitwood, 1995, pp.139).

Ten years later, within an investigation on quality of life in dementia, Fukushima and colleagues (2005) gathered information from family caregivers about changes that they had observed within their family member with dementia. Caregivers noted that although their family member had initially struggled with the difficulties posed by their condition, they developed, over time, an acceptance of dementia. Family members were subsequently described as quiet and calm, showing relaxed behaviours that had not been seen previously by family, such as singing and dancing. They were seen to focus more than before on living life in the present, showing more interest and open-mindedness, seeming more aware of the importance of their relationships, and demonstrating gratitude and sensitivity towards others. Fukushima *et al.* (2005, p.33) concluded that, whilst participants' positive personality styles had been sustained in the presence of dementia, other 'new aspects of their humanity were nurtured under the condition'.

Research into the experience of spirituality for people living with dementia has identified that although the condition can challenge faith and spiritual practice, people have also been able to find a deep sense of meaning in their life and in their dementia – for example, by experiencing dementia as purposeful (providing an important lesson or spiritual test) or enhancing their faith (Dalby, Sperlinger and Boddington, 2012; Phinney, 2011; Snyder, 2003; Stuckey *et al.*, 2002).

A recent review of qualitative research on positive experiences whilst living with dementia (Wolverson, Clarke and Moniz-Cook, 2015) identified a theme of growing and transcending, in which individuals with dementia had similarly described gaining a kind of spiritual wisdom through living with dementia. Furthermore, individuals explained how dementia had provided them with opportunities for self-discovery and helping others, and had enabled them to develop a broader view on life. However, within original studies, these experiences tended to have been interpreted within frameworks of maintaining spirituality, coping and staying positive in the face of dementia. Although these interpretations are valid, it is important to question whether traditionally negative discourses and assumptions surrounding dementia may limit the conclusions that are drawn when listening to the perspectives of people living with it – is it only possible to cope with the condition or can some people in fact grow with it?

In an attempt to explore further the subjective experience of growth within the context of dementia, we conducted a study (Patterson, 2015), which directly enquired about participants' experiences of positive and meaningful changes since living with dementia, and explored how participants had made sense of these changes. Nine older people living with dementia in the community were interviewed, and a qualitative analysis led to the development of two key themes: *Moving Forward* and *Living in the Now*.

The first theme, 'Moving Forward', reflected a sense of forward momentum and continuity in people's lives, but also, crucially, a sense of evolution. This evolution meant that, more than ever, participants were motivated to seek out positive emotions and experiences, because, as one person explained this was 'the difference [that] growing old makes. You don't want to waste time on things you can't do anything about, and also you don't want to be unhappy too much' (p.84).

Dementia offered new opportunities for developing and utilising the values and traits that participants had held throughout their lives – for example, by bringing a sense of openness, support or humour to others who were living with the condition. In other cases, new traits and values were developed or uncovered within the person. For example, some felt that they were now able to speak their own mind, had shifted their focus in life to concentrate upon love and relationships, or felt a greater sense of compassion for others' difficulties. As one individual explained: 'I've always been compassionate, but compassionate in a very thin way... I didn't really pay attention to a lot of the things going on that didn't concern me... [Now] my compassion's got bigger' (p.167).

Participants' experiences suggested that they were continuing to learn about life and about themselves and had the capacity to continue to develop in positive and meaningful ways. As one person explained: 'That's how I look at my dementia as well. It's a volcano that's there, it's dangerous, but at the bottom of that, there's a fertile land, that you can grow and you can expand' (p.87).

Alongside this theme of moving forward, there was also a sense that participants were focused upon 'Living in the Now'. Within this theme, participants remained aware of the future threats posed by their dementia, but chose not to dwell upon these: "There's people I've spoken to and they've said the sort of things, "Oh I think it will get worse next week" or "just forget all of that", choosing instead to "just look at today, you know, not tomorrow"' (p.167).

Whilst the uncertain future and the prospect of their condition advancing were frightening, it enabled people to attribute more importance and significance to the present day. Participants felt *'lucky'* with the lives that they lived in the present: '[It] makes you realise, shall we say, to be satisfied with what you've got.' Living with dementia now motivated people to do the things that they wanted to do *now*, and to *live* each day:

> I do things now. I don't procrastinate about them. I don't say 'Well, I could do that tomorrow, I could do that that day and there, there, there. I do it now because I don't know what's going to happen to me when I wake up. (p.168)

'Edward' – a case illustration

'Edward' (a pseudonym) initially explained that he was not sure how much he could contribute to a positive psychology study, as he did not have many positive things to say about life with dementia. However, what he proceeded to describe was a very thoughtful and moving account of how his diagnosis of dementia had facilitated a process of reflection, a changing perspective on what is meaningful in life, and a commitment to self-improvement in order to pursue what is most important.

Being diagnosed with dementia had caused Edward to reflect heavily upon how he had lived his life thus far, and at times, he was critical of choices he had made about relating to others across the years. Edward's main concern was that he could have shown more warmth within his interpersonal life: 'I feel guilty that I've probably not...been as warm to people as – to the family – as I might have been...a bit more compassion, and a bit more love, won't go amiss.'

At other times, Edward's thinking was orientated towards the future. Due to his awareness of the progressive nature of dementia, these thoughts were frightening on occasion, but, overall, Edward explained that he did not often perceive the future as overly bleak: 'I naturally started thinking, well, what...what might become of myself, you know – not necessarily in too negative a way...because I don't think it is all that negative to be about it really.' Instead, this future-focus appeared to have helped Edward to establish in what position he would like to be in the future – specifically, what kind of relationships he would like to have with his friends and family in the years to come. In fact, Edward later identified that this was more than a simple preference or desire: 'I think wanting to is a bit glib, I think it's more...it's a need.' This was a need to be in a position where he could be secure in the knowledge that he was liked and loved by those close to him: '[A] need for me, to want that warmth, from me family as well. Which sounds a little bit of a selfish thing but...I want my family to like me and love me.'

Edward appeared to have come to the conclusion that he wanted to be a person who prioritised love, emotions and relationships: '[L]ove and affection, yes, are the priorities.' This was because having dementia had made him realise that it wasn't the things that he had done or achieved that were important; what really mattered in life were the relationships he had with other people: '[T]he balance has shifted, and the...the other side of the coin, is the important side. The relationships. That's what's important... It was always really important what you'd done, who you were – [that] becomes less important.' He consequently took active steps towards engaging with others – for example, by adding more warmth to his interactions with family or by making sure to share a few words with people he met in his day-to-day life:

> I try to talk to more people, you know, always being aware of people, trying to be...just you know...trying to generally be more aware of the people that are around me and to dare just to exchange words with them.

As Edward described, making these changes was difficult, as he felt that his natural tendency was to be somewhat introverted, and to focus upon the scientific and the logical instead of the relational. He consequently had to '*battle*' against his own personality in order to make the changes that were important to him: 'I get in the way of it, I think. My personality gets in the way of it... [It's] not always easy to achieve, but, [it]'s what I want.' Edward explained that throughout his life, he had been aware that these were changes that needed to be made. Dementia appeared to be a critical stimulus that prompted him to consider these changes and to begin putting them into action: 'I've done quite a bit of analysis, you know. I think it [diagnosis] forces you to do that.' He acknowledged that he was a *changing*, not completely *changed* man. But he believed that developing the emotional and relational side of the self was important to well-being in general, and particularly important in enabling him to live well with a condition that posed threats to his self-identity and painted an uncertain future:

> I was aware of me inwardness, and...I knew that was a problem...my inwardness is more of a problem to me condition, and I cannot afford to be inward-looking with this condition. I have to be outward-looking, if I'm going to get the benefits, or, to counter, in any way I can, the condition that I've got.

Edward had always held an awareness of what was important and meaningful in life, but living with a progressive illness, meant that he was motivated to pursue these now:

> I need to be more open for the condition, and I need to be more open for me own personality. The two have come together to form a bond there... I no longer can sit back and think oh I can do that tomorrow, I can be more open with people. Now I've got to do it. Now I've got to try and be more open. Because that's going to help me as well.

IMPLICATIONS

The findings of this study highlight key points in relation to growth and well-being amongst people living with dementia. First, they attest to the notion that people continue to learn, grow and develop throughout the course of their lives and that people living with dementia need not be an exception to this. Second, the findings highlight the possibility that the processes underpinning growth in the context of a significant illness may also be applicable to people living with a condition such as dementia. The experiences of some participants suggested that the presence of dementia did more than simply not preclude growth – in some instances, it stimulated growth in new and unexpected ways.

These findings lend support to Weiss's (2014) suggestion that growth can be created through an interplay between life-span development and post-traumatic forms of growth. It was clear from participants' narratives that their subjective experiences were not entirely shaped by dementia, and that there was not always one singular 'catalyst' for growth amongst individuals who were growing older, living with dementia, and experiencing other life events along the way. Finally, the study has implications for our understanding of how well-being and quality of life might be experienced and enhanced amongst individuals living with dementia. They indicate that dementia is not solely a loss-based experience, and it is therefore not sufficient for us to only consider how individuals can be supported to *maintain* their identity, relationships and ways of functioning. In addition, we must also consider the possibility that well-being may be facilitated by *further developing* these aspects of an individual's personal and social identities, or even by *discovering new* aspects of identity and new possibilities for life. As Orbach (1996, p.27) reflects, a person with dementia must be respected for 'what she (or he) once was, and also for what she, mysteriously, still is, as well as what she may become'.

CONCLUSIONS

The literature presented here lends support to the notion that growth may be a viable pathway to well-being amongst people living with dementia. However, current theory and research relating to growth and well-being is varied, with numerous ideas, arguments and inconsistencies throughout the literature – quite possibly because growth and well-being are multi-faceted constructs. In particular, theory and research relating to growth amongst people living with dementia is clearly lacking. We need to understand more about *how* growth may be nurtured in the context of dementia, how far it is subject to cognitive ability and how it may be linked to the well-being of people living with the condition. We need to be wary of assuming that dementia is entirely associated with loss and decline on a subjective level; we must ask directly about growth experiences and recognise them to be genuine where they do occur, taking care to understand them in context. Further research is therefore needed to examine the impact of the social environment and how growth amongst people living with dementia might be inhibited or nurtured in the presence of certain social conditions.

Despite the limitations in the literature, we can tentatively draw out some hypotheses about processes that may be important in fostering a link between growth and heightened well-being in dementia. For some people, growth may represent an important coping strategy that helps to maintain or improve well-being – for example, by finding meaning or benefits in their situation, or fostering a sense of personal resilience to cope with challenges posed by the condition. In other cases, growth through ageing may enhance well-being by supporting older people with dementia to develop a coherent sense of self (Erikson, 1963) and an acceptance of self and the life that has been lived (Tornstam, 2011). Growth may also involve the development or expansion of new perspectives – for example, reaching new heights of spirituality and connectedness, experiencing a broader sense of identity, or perhaps focusing upon the needs of others (Reed, 1991), a process that has been described in the literature around dementia-related activism (e.g. Bartlett, 2014a, 2014b). Perhaps for some people, growth in later life and dementia may be more of an experiential, *felt* sense rather than based on cognitive appraisals, as described by Bauer and Park (2010). For others still, growth may lead to changes in attitude and behaviour that impact positively on an individual's personal, social or existential well-being. For example, in the case of Edward described earlier, living with dementia caused him to re-consider his perspectives and priorities, leading him to re-focus his time and energy on what was most important to him.

Pathways to growth are likely to be multiple, varied and shaped by the individuals who tread them. As 'Fred' (a pseudonym) noted, 'This [dementia] has been my road to Damascus. It's been such a road. It's opened so many avenues, so many pathways, that sometimes I can't pick what pathway I want to go down' (Patterson *et al.*, 2015).

New paths may be opened up for personal growth through dementia, whilst other paths may be extended as people grow throughout their life-span. There is much still to learn and we can only discover more by listening to the subjective experiences of each individual and by opening our own minds towards stories that depict not just endings but new beginnings.

REFERENCES

Baltes, P.B. and Staudinger, U.M. (2000) 'Wisdom: A metaheuristic (pragmatic) to orchestrate mind and virtue towards excellence.' *American Psychologist 55*, 122–136.

Barskova, T. and Oesterreich, R. (2009) 'Post-traumatic growth in people living with a serious medical condition and its relations to physical and mental health: A systematic review.' *Disability and Rehabilitation 31*(21), 1709–1733.

Bartlett, R. (2014a) 'The emergent modes of dementia activism.' *Ageing and Society 34*(4), 623–644.

Bartlett, R. (2014b) 'Citizenship in action: The lived experiences of citizens with dementia who campaign for social change.' *Disability and Society 29*(8), 1291–1304.

Bauer, J.J. and Park, S.W. (2010) 'Growth is Not Just for the Young: Growth Narratives, Eudaimonic Resilience, and the Ageing Self.' In P.S. Fry and C.L. Keyes (eds) *New Frontiers in Resilient Ageing: Life-Strengths and Well-being in Late Life.* New York, NY: Cambridge University Press.

Braam, A.W., Bramsen, I., van Tilburg, T.G., van der Ploeg, H.M. and Deeg, D.J.H. (2006) 'Cosmic transcendence and framework of meaning in life: Patterns among older adults in the Netherlands.' *Journal of Gerontology 61B*(3), S121–S128.

Bryden, C. (2005) *Dancing with Dementia: My Story of Living Positively with Dementia.* London: Jessica Kingsley Publishers.

Carver C.S. (1998) 'Resilience and thriving: Issues, models, and linkages.' *Journal of Social Issues 54*(2), 245–266.

Dalby, P., Sperlinger, D. J. and Boddington, S. (2012) 'The lived experience of spirituality and dementia in older people living with mild to moderate dementia.' *Dementia 11*(1), 75–94.

Davis, C.G., Nolen-Hoeksema, S. and Larson, J. (1998) 'Making sense of loss and benefiting from the experience: Two construals of meaning.' *Journal of Personality and Social Psychology 75*(2), 561–574.

Deci, E.L. and Ryan, R.M. (2008) 'Hedonia, eudaimonia, and well-being: An introduction.' *Journal of Happiness Studies 9*(1), 1–11.

Erikson, E.H. (1963) *Childhood and Society.* New York: W.W. Norton & Company, Inc.

Erikson, E.H. and Erikson, J.M. (1997) *The Life Cycle Completed* (extended version with new chapters on the ninth stage of development). New York, NY: W.W. Norton & Company, Inc.

Eve, P. and Kangas, M. (2015) 'Posttraumatic growth following trauma: Is growth accelerated or a reflection of cognitive maturation?' *The Humanistic Psychologist 43*(4), 354–370.

Filipp, S.H. (1999) 'A Three-stage Model of Coping with Loss and Trauma.' In A. Maercker, M. Schützwohl and Z. Solomon (eds) *Posttraumatic Stress Disorder: A Life-span Developmental Perspective.* Seattle, WA: Hogrefe & Huber.

Fredrickson, B.L. and Losada, M.F. (2005) 'Positive affect and the complex dynamics of human flourishing.' *American Psychologist 60*(7), 678–686.

Fromm, E. (1955) *The Sane Society.* New York, NY: Fawcett Prier Books.

Fukushima, T., Nagahata, K., Ishibashi, N., Takahashi, Y. and Moriyama, M. (2005) 'Quality of life from the viewpoint of patients with dementia in Japan: Nurturing through an acceptance of dementia by patients, their families and care professionals.' *Health and Social Care in the Community 13*(1) 30–37.

Gillen, G. (2005) 'Positive consequences of surviving a stroke.' *American Journal of Occupational Therapy 59*(3), 346–350.

Hefferon, K., Grealy, M. and Mutrie, N. (2009) 'Post-traumatic growth and life threatening physical illness: A systematic review of the qualitative literature.' *British Journal of Health Psychology 14*(2), 343–378.

Helgeson, V.S., Reynolds, K.A. and Tomich, P.L. (2006) 'A meta-analytic review of benefit finding and growth.' *Journal of Consulting and Clinical Psychology* 74(5), 797–816.

Hemingway, E. (2012) *A Farewell to Arms* (original work published 1929). New York, NY: Scribner.

Hobfoll, S.E., Hall, B.J., Canetti-Nisim, D., Galea, S., Johnson, R.J. and Palmieri, P.A. (2007) 'Refining our understanding of traumatic growth in the face of terrorism: Moving from meaning cognitions to doing what is meaningful.' *Applied Psychology* 56(3), 345–366.

Joseph, S. and Linley, P.A. (2005) 'Positive adjustment to threatening events: An organismic valuing theory of growth through adversity.' *Review of General Psychology* 9(3), 262–280.

Joseph, S. and Linley, P.A. (2008) 'Psychological Assessment of Growth Following Adversity: A Review.' In S. Joseph and P.A. Linley (eds) *Trauma, Recovery, and Growth: Positive Psychological Perspectives on Posttraumatic Stress*. New Jersey, NJ: John Wiley & Sons, Inc.

Jung, C. (1970) *The Structure and Dynamics of the Psyche*. New York, NY: Pantheon Books, Inc.

Kampman, H., Hefferon, K., Wilson, M. and Beale, J. (2015) '"I can do things now that people thought were impossible, actually, things that I thought were impossible": A meta-synthesis of the qualitative findings on posttraumatic growth and severe physical injury.' *Canadian Psychology/Psychologie Canadienne* 56(3), 283–294.

Keyes, C.L. (2002) 'The mental health continuum: From languishing to flourishing in life.' *Journal of Health and Social Behavior* 43(2), 207–222.

Kitwood, T. (1990) 'The dialectics of dementia: with particular reference to Alzheimer's disease.' *Ageing and Society* 10(2), 177–196.

Kitwood, T. (1995) 'Positive long-term changes in dementia: Some preliminary observations.' *Journal of Mental Health* 4(2), 133–144.

Koltko-Rivera, M.E. (2006) 'Rediscovering the later version of Maslow's hierarchy of needs: Self-transcendence and opportunities for theory, research, and unification.' *Review of General Psychology* 10(4), 302–317.

Koutrouli, N., Anagnostopoulos, F. and Potamianos, G. (2012) 'Posttraumatic stress disorder and posttraumatic growth in breast cancer patients: A systematic review.' *Women and Health* 52(5), 503–516.

Maslow, A.H. (1954) *Motivation and Personality*. New York, NY: Harper & Row.

Maslow, A.H. (1969) 'The farther reaches of human nature.' *Journal of Transpersonal Psychology* 1(1), 1–9.

McFarland, C. and Alvaro, C. (2000) 'The impact of motivation on temporal comparisons: Coping with traumatic events by perceiving personal growth.' *Journal of Personality and Social Psychology* 79(3), 327–343.

Montoya-Juarez, R. *et al.* (2013) 'Psychological responses of terminally ill patients who are experiencing suffering: A qualitative study.' *International Journal of Nursing Studies* 50(1), 53–62.

Mystakidou, K., Tsilika, E., Parpa, E., Galanos, A. and Vlahos, L. (2008) 'Post-traumatic growth in advanced cancer patients receiving palliative care.' *British Journal of Health Psychology 13*(4), 633–646.

Orbach, A. (1996) *Not Too Late: Psychotherapy and Ageing.* London: Jessica Kingsley Publishers.

O'Sullivan, G., Hocking, C. and Spence, D. (2014) 'Dementia: The need for attitudinal change.' *Dementia 13*(4), 483–497.

Pakenham, K.I. (2007) 'The nature of benefit finding in multiple sclerosis (MS).' *Psychology, Health and Medicine 12*(2), 190–196.

Park, C.L. and Folkman, S. (1997) 'Meaning in the context of stress and coping.' *Review of General Psychology 1*(2), 115.

Paterson, B.L. (2001) 'The shifting perspectives model of chronic illness.' *Journal of Nursing Scholarship 33*(1), 21–26.

Paterson, K. (2015) 'Responses to dementia: A qualitative exploration of self and others.' (Unpublished doctoral thesis), University of Hull, Hull.

Peacock, S. *et al.* (2009) 'The positive aspects of the caregiving journey with dementia: Using a strengths-based perspective to reveal opportunities.' *Journal of Applied Gerontology 29*(5), 640–659.

Phinney, A. (2011) 'Horizons of meaning in dementia: Retained and shifting narratives.' *Journal of Religion, Spirituality and Aging 23*(3), 254–268.

Read, S., Braam, A.W., Lyyra, T.M. and Deeg, D. J. (2014) 'Do negative life events promote gerotranscendence in the second half of life?' *Aging and Mental Health 18*(1), 117–124.

Reed, P.G. (1991) 'Toward a nursing theory of self-transcendence: Deductive reformulation using developmental theories.' *Advances in Nursing Science 13*(4), 64–77.

Robinson, L. Clare, L. and Evans, K. (2005) 'Making sense of dementia and adjusting to loss: Psychological reactions to a diagnosis of dementia in couples.' *Aging and Mental Health 9*(4), 337–347.

Rogers, C.R. (1951) *Client-centered Therapy: Its Current Practice, Implications and Theory.* London: Constable & Co. Ltd.

Rogers, C.R. (1959) 'A Theory of Therapy, Personality, and Interpersonal Relationships, as Developed in the Client-centered Framework.' In S. Koch (ed.) *Psychology: A Study of a Science. Study 1, Volume 3: Formulations of the Person and the Social Context.* New York, NY: McGraw-Hill.

Ryff, C.D. and Keyes, C.L.M. (1995) 'The structure of psychological well-being revisited.' *Journal of Personality and Social Psychology 69*(4), 719–727.

Ryff, C.D. and Singer, B. (2003) 'Flourishing Under Fire: Resilience as a Prototype of Challenged Thriving.' In C.L.M. Keyes and J. Haidt (eds) *Flourishing: Positive Psychology and the Life Well-lived.* Washington DC: American Psychological Association.

Ryff, C.D. and Singer, B.H. (2008) 'Know thyself and become what you are: A eudaimonic approach to psychological well-being.' *Journal of Happiness Studies 9*(1), 13–39.

Sawyer, A., Ayers, S. and Field, A.P. (2010) 'Posttraumatic growth and adjustment among individuals with cancer or HIV/AIDS: A meta-analysis.' *Clinical Psychology Review 30*(4), 436–447.

Snyder, L. (2003) 'Satisfactions and challenges in spiritual faith and practice for persons with dementia.' *Dementia 2*(3), 299–313.

Stuckey, J.C., Post, S.G., Ollerton, S., FallCreek, S.J. and Whitehouse, P.J. (2002) 'Alzheimer's disease, religion, and the ethics of respect for spirituality: A community dialogue.' *Alzheimer's Care Today 3*(3), 199–207.

Tang, S.T., Lin, K.C., Chen, J.S., Chang, W.C., Hsieh, C.H. and Chou, W.C. (2015) 'Threatened with death but growing: Changes in and determinants of posttraumatic growth over the dying process for Taiwanese terminally ill cancer patients.' *Psycho-Oncology 24*(2), 147–154.

Taylor, S.E. (1983) 'Adjustment to threatening events: A theory of cognitive adaptation.' *American Psychologist 38*(11), 1161–1173.

Tedeschi, R.G. and Calhoun, L.G. (1996) 'The Posttraumatic Growth Inventory: Measuring the positive legacy of trauma.' *Journal of Traumatic Stress 9*(3), 455–471.

Tedeschi, R.G. and Calhoun, L.G. (2004). 'Posttraumatic growth: Conceptual foundations and empirical evidence.' *Psychological Inquiry 15*(1), 1–18.

Tomich, P.L., and Helgeson, V.S. (2004) 'Is finding something good in the bad always good? Benefit finding among women with breast cancer.' *Health Psychology 23*(1), 16–23.

Tornstam, L. (1989) 'Gero-transcendence: A reformulation of the disengagement theory.' *Ageing Clinical and Experimental Research 1*(1), 55–63.

Tornstam, L. (1999) 'Transcendence in later life.' *Generations 23*(4), 10–14.

Tornstam, L. (2005) *Gerotranscendence: A Developmental Theory of Positive Ageing.* New York, NY: Springer Publishing Company, Inc.

Tornstam, L. (2011) 'Maturing into gerotranscendence.' *Journal of Transpersonal Psychology 43*, 166–180.

Wadensten, B. (2005) 'Introducing older people to the theory of gerotranscendence.' *Journal of Advanced Nursing 52*(4), 381–388.

Weiss, T. (2002) 'Posttraumatic growth in women with breast cancer and their husbands: An intersubjective validation study.' *Journal of Psychosocial Oncology 20*(2), 65–80.

Weiss, T. (2014) Personal transformation posttraumatic growth and gerotranscendence.' *Journal of Humanistic Psychology 54*(2), 203–226.

Wolverson, E.L., Clarke, C. and Moniz-Cook, E.D. (2015) 'Living positively with dementia: A systematic review and synthesis of the qualitative literature.' *Aging and Mental Health*. DOI :10.1080/13607863.2015.1052777

Zoellner, T. and Maercker, A. (2006) 'Posttraumatic growth in clinical psychology—a critical review and introduction of a two component model.' *Clinical Psychology Review 26*(5), 626–653.

Chapter 8

CREATIVITY AND DEMENTIA

John Killick

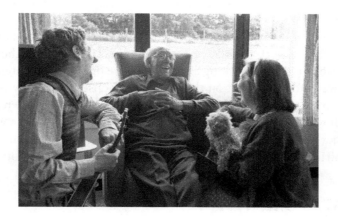

INTRODUCTION

In this chapter we shall first of all look at creativity, its nature and its
role in the lives of people living with dementia. Whereas many might
assume that the cognitive changes associated with dementia would
inevitably impair a person's capacity for creativity, this chapter aims to
demonstrate that creative activities remain possible and can provide
important ways of making meaning and increasing well-being. I
have limited myself mainly to a discussion of artistic aspects of the

subject. This will involve a consideration of such concepts as process, the moment and flow, and these will be explored through instances of drama, dance and poetry. I shall conclude with examining the ideas of valuing and evaluating creativity.

I begin with two stories from my own experience: Whilst travelling on a train, I overheard a young boy (I guessed he was about seven years old) in the seat in front of me reacting to someone walking down the carriage holding a bunch of daffodils. 'They don't smell when they have honey on', he said. A few days earlier I had been walking through the lounge area of a dementia care unit on a sunny afternoon, when a woman (I guessed she would be in her eighties) called out to me: 'If you're not careful, you'll spend your days in the land of striped sunshine.'

I suggest that what these two declarations have in common is that neither of them employs the logical properties of language. They are both exclamations and imaginative responses to experience. I am aware that in putting these two incidents side by side I am running the risk of being accused of comparing a child to someone with dementia. Of course, in many ways the two individuals are very different, but they are alike in this respect: in order to articulate their perceptions, they both make use of creative thinking and the creative properties of language.

If we go on to reflect on the kind of responses evoked by the two statements, we will probably have to agree that the most likely reaction to the boy is one of delight and enthusiasm, whereas that to the woman is for her to be ignored or scorned with such comments as 'she's away with fairies'. Yet, to my mind, she is revealing hidden poetic potential.

WHAT IS CREATIVITY?

Creativity is a word with wide connotations. Almost any activity can be considered to have creative aspects if approached with an open-minded spirit (i.e. being curious and ready to entertain new ideas). Work, sport, hobbies and domestic chores can all be approached in this frame of mind. There are many theories of creativity within positive psychology (Kaufman and Sternberg, 2010). Broadly, creativity is seen as a process (often a mental process) in which a person (often seen as a certain type of person with a trait or flair for creativity) creates a product that is both novel (surprising, unusual or original) and useful or adaptive (Peterson and Seligman, 2004) within a specific social context.

THE CREATIVE PROCESS

Creativity is often conceptualised as a mental process and there has been extensive work exploring the relationship between creativity and intelligence. The research suggests that, although a certain level of intellectual capacity is the bedrock for creativity to be demonstrated, beyond that threshold it can be exercised with considerable freedom (Barron and Harrington, 1981). Cognitive abilities such as divergent thinking (Guilford, 1967) and divided attention (Peterson and Seligman, 2004), which are often considered to be problematic for people living with dementia, have been cited as important to creative thinking. Research exploring neurobiological processes and creativity is still at a very early stage; however, the dominant role of the right hemisphere in creative thinking is widely recognised. Given that creativity involves the integration of ideas, it is likely to involve diverse brain regions and especially those in the frontal lobes (Takeuchi *et al.*, 2010). However, such scientific investigations of creativity appear at odds with the lay understanding of the concept, for many people would argue that what distinguishes a creative person is their disposition, not their intelligence.

THE CREATIVE PERSON

A common assumption is that creativity is a special trait that some people exhibit and others are denied access to in their daily lives. We may often hear people claim that they do not possess a capacity to exercise creativity and reject any opportunities that present themselves to put this belief to the test. A creative person, according to Sternberg and Lubart's (1999) investment theory of creativity, is not just someone who possesses 'raw talent' but a person with the ability to see problems that need solutions and who has an openness to experience as well as a sense of agency and motivation.

Whilst not denying that some individuals can develop their talents, artistic and otherwise, to a high level, Csikszentmihalyi's systems model of creativity (1998) conceptualises creativity as a systemic rather than an individualistic process. The model suggests that creativity is an interaction between a creative individual who has become immersed in a field and comes up with an original idea and an audience who may be ambivalent about accepting the idea. So, according to this theory, families and cultures can foster creativity and support creative endeavours, irrespective of the particular talents of the individual undertaking a creative act.

THE PRODUCT

Creativity has also been measured in terms of its product or end result. Creative products are often defined as novel and adaptive; they are considered to make a positive contribution to the life of the person and of others.

An issue that arises time and again is that of process versus product. What has mattered to artists and the public over the centuries and across cultures is the finished 'work of art'. The court painter or composer has been judged on the quality (and perhaps quantity) of the works created. However, the late 20th century saw increased fascination with the ways artworks are created, the inspiration that goes into them and the techniques used to realise the vision of the artist. This shows no sign of abating. At the time of writing, for example, the singer/songwriter P.J. Harvey in London is creating an album in public – the Artangel project involves a specially equipped studio where, over a month, Harvey rehearses and records, while spectators pay for the privilege of observing from the other side of a one-way glass wall and listen in through speakers. *The Guardian* article on this unique event (Searle, 2015) begins with the sentence 'Mostly, the creative process is boring.' No doubt our present obsession with process arises, at least in part, from the mystery inherent in creativity.

In the case of projects with people with dementia, however, the process of creativity is probably the most significant aspect, for reasons I shall go on to outline below. In the context of creativity and dementia, amongst the aspects I can identify as important are the following:

- It must give pleasure for its own sake.

- There is a making process involved, which may result in an outcome (a poem or a painting or a performance).

- It can provide an opportunity for celebration.

- It must be expressive of the person or the group.

- It can be one of the ways to experience 'flow' or optimum experience, whether there is an end-product or not.

In other words, it has the capacity by various means to enhance life.

CREATIVITY AND AGEING

Later life is often characterised as a time when productivity declines. We might be led to believe that a person's creative juices simply dry up as they age! However, there is no evidence that creativity declines with age at a trait level, but rather research suggests that individual differences in creativity tend to be fairly stable over time (Peterson and Seligman, 2004). Others have argued that there can often be a resurgence in creative expression, both qualitatively and quantitatively, in later life (Lindauer, 1993). Some report a burst of creativity in later life, a 'swan song' whereby creative people seem to develop striking late styles and become even more capable of expressing deep thoughts and feelings (e.g. see Arnheim, 1986; Dormandy, 2000; Einstein, 1956; Lindauer, 1992, 1993, 2003). Indeed, there are many examples of famous artists approaching death who became motivated to produce incredible final works as their creative legacy. A case in point is Matisse, who, at the age of 74 and after battling cancer, found himself bed-bound and unable to paint or sculpt anymore yet went on to prolifically produce his well-known 'cut outs'. Creativity in later life may not be restricted to those who only displayed it in earlier life; it is possible that creativity could increase as part of the life-cycle, where turning inward for renewal or perhaps even difficult or personally challenging circumstances might act as catalysts for creativity (Peterson and Seligman, 2004).

Creative concepts and techniques throw down a challenge to us as we get older, as we become more reliant upon our habits and routines to set the parameters for living. Chance and the unexpected, the playful and the experimental, can bring a new joyfulness into our lives. As such, it has been suggested that creativity might facilitate successful ageing by encouraging the development of problem-solving skills, motivation and deeper self-understanding, which could in turn help people to cope more readily with challenges and problems they may face in later life. Fisher, Bradley and Specht (1999) conducted a qualitative study of 36 older people involved in arts projects and reported that for these people creative activity provided a sense of competence, purpose and growth.

Similarly, in a ten-year longitudinal study, Dawson and Baller (1972) found that older people involved in creative arts live longer, healthier lives than age-matched cohorts.

WHY PEOPLE WITH DEMENTIA?

People with cognitive impairment predominantly fall into the category of older persons, and providing them with continued, respectful occupation and stimulation should rank high on anyone's list of priorities. Added to this, the restrictions laid upon them by their condition and their carers' reactions to this, as well as the fact that they are surrounded by stigma, means they must be given every chance to demonstrate that their personhood is intact and their remaining talents are valued. Creative activities offer the chance to achieve this.

It may be that people living with dementia have a special capacity for artistic experience. This could be partly due to a recovery of innocence of response, and, in some instances, of the development of a degree of disinhibition. Certainly, the fact that the arts are not dependent upon intellectual capacity, and in the case of some art-forms, of verbal abilities, is an advantage. But if we consider all the changes that are happening to people, often unprecedented and apparently irreversible, it is incontestable that people living with dementia should have significant means of expressing themselves, if only as a means of processing the changes they are undergoing.

Agnes Houston, a younger person with dementia in Scotland, is keenly aware of what the arts can offer someone in her position:

> I wanted to find out if I was artistic. Creativity's an aspect I wanted to explore. Being able to feel out of the box is what I'm picking up. It will happen. It's a bit like waiting for Christmas. You know it's coming, but as a child you don't exactly know when. It's a nice feeling.

THE IDEA OF THE MOMENT

The reason why creative process takes centre stage in dementia is that memory-loss creates windows of opportunity, which may be small but can be capitalised upon. We are looking here at concentrated periods that will be discontinuous, and this makes it difficult, if not impossible, to contemplate an aggregated whole. Each session of creativity may be discrete and valued for its own sake. So, intensity is possible even if consistency is unlikely to be achieved. It is a common observation that people with dementia live in the moment, so the strategy has to be to fill as many of those moments with as much meaningfulness as possible.

THE IDEA OF FLOW

If 'the moment' is accepted as the basic unit of creative provision for people with dementia, there arises the need to explore the various ways in which it can be utilised. One of the most fruitful of these approaches may be that of flow – a subjective state that people report when they become totally absorbed in a task or an activity for its own sake and that results in a sense of satisfaction and losing track of time (Csikszentmihalyi, 1990). Nakamura and Csikszentmihalyi (2005) described the characteristics people display when experiencing flow as:

* a reduced awareness of the external environment

* awareness being intensely focused on the task and the present moment

* a reduction in self-consciousness

* a lack of awareness of the passage of time

* a strong sense of control and achievement.

When an individual is in flow they operate at their full capacity and thus flow has been described as an 'optimal experience' because individuals are fully involved in the present moment. The case for linking the concepts of flow and the moment together has been made eloquently by Nakamura and Csziksentmihalyi (2005, p.102): 'Although it seems clear that flow serves as a buffer against adversity and prevents pathology, its major contribution to the quality of life consists in endowing momentary experience with value.'

Experiencing flow encourages a person to persist and return to activities because of the experiential rewards it promises (Nakamura and Csikszentmihalyi, 2005). Thus, flow activities encourage mastery and achievement and provide an opportunity for people to develop and improve skills as well as achieve satisfaction and a sense of accomplishment. In this way creativity contributes to well-being in 'social, emotional, and functional' ways (Forgeard *et al.*, 2011, p.81) through facilitating accomplishment, engagement, expression and meaning.

Kate Allan (2008, p.24), in one of the few articles to link flow with dementia, poses the question: 'If achieving a state of flow can have a beneficial general effect on mental functioning for individuals without dementia, could it have a similar positive effect on those affected by the condition?'

An individual can find flow in almost any activity because flow is based upon subjective challenges and skills. In order to experience flow, the task we are engaged in must achieve a balance between the challenges of the task and the abilities of the participant. For a person to be motivated to complete a task, they must find it enjoyable. Flow activities can be done alone or with others. Crucially, flow is also a dynamic experience between the person and their social environment.

As such, people can experience flow in ostensibly mundane day-to-day pursuits (e.g. household tasks). Being able to continue engaging in ordinary activities of daily living might therefore assist some people with dementia to experience flow, but it seems likely that for others engagement in creative challenges may increase their capacity for having and benefiting from this experience. I suggest that it may be possible to view the comments of the participants in the three projects described later in this chapter as reactions to occasions when they experienced flow in their various creative activities, which in the context of living with dementia may prove very challenging. Their voices carry powerful implications about the experience of creativity in dementia, but there is also an urgent need for further research in this area. We can only speculate how the lives of people with dementia and their caregivers might be enriched if they were regularly offered opportunities of this kind through the design and provision of activities or environments designed to foster flow, or by attempting to assist individuals in finding flow in their daily experiences. One can posit a situation where a carer and a person with the condition could form a partnership to explore flow activities, creating opportunities for positive emotional experiences throughout their lives together.

PORTRAITS

So how might we ensure that people living with dementia are provided with supportive, reinforcing and open environments that foster their creativity? According to a systems model (Csikszentmihalyi, 1998), creativity is fostered by inclusive social environments where threats to survival are low and where there is a surplus of mental and physical energy. This is a particular challenge for people with dementia, who may often find themselves in social environments where they either feel excluded or where close and critical supervision stifles creativity. The best way to illustrate the possibilities of a creative approach to dementia care is to give some examples of the arts in action and the lived experiences connected with them. I have chosen three art-forms for in-depth descriptions: 1) a drama project exploiting elements of humour to draw out the creativity of participants; 2) dance as an enhancement of in-the-body experiences; and 3) poetry as a means of harnessing the natural verbal expressiveness of individuals.

1. ELDERFLOWERS AND HUMOUR

Hearts & Minds is one of the longest-established arts schemes in the UK working with groups in hospitals and other institutions throughout Scotland. It has been successfully practising for 13 years. It has two strands: 'Clowndoctors', targeting sick children; and 'Elderflowers', working with people with dementia. At the time of writing the organisation is working in 27 locations, covering 14 local authorities and employing 21 clowns across both schemes. In this humour project, I have observed how laughter is the key to unlocking creative communication:

- Humour is used as a 'calling card' – playfulness breaks down the barriers and allows connections to be established.

- Humour modulates into serious conversations on subjects of interest and concern to individuals and then, seemingly effortlessly, becomes jokey again.

- The highly developed sensitivities of the Elderflower actors to the general atmosphere and the individual psyches of the patients (to them 'ladies and gentlemen') ensures flexibility of response.

- The personalities of the Elderflowers seem to take on a new dimension of openness and attractiveness when the personas of sympathetic clowns are adopted.

- The Elderflowers fail all the time, which puts them on the level with those with whom they are interacting (that is what makes them open and vulnerable and responsive).

- Lastly, the project is meeting the challenge of communicating and relating to those individuals who pose the greatest difficulties – a challenge that other arts projects designed for people with dementia often avoid.

The Elderflowers Project demonstrates a general principle of creative relationships with people with dementia: that playfulness is not only to be valued for its own sake but is an enabling tool for establishing connections and instituting change and development. As Stephen Nachmanovitch puts it in his remarkable book *Free Play*:

> This is the evolutionary value of play – play makes us flexible. By reinterpreting reality and begetting novelty, we keep from becoming rigid. Play enables us to rearrange our capacities and our very identity so that they can be used in unforeseen ways. (Nachmanovitch, 1990, p.43)

Probably the most important overall characteristic that Elderflowers' practice illustrates is that they are not performing for the participants, but attempting to draw out qualities from them – characteristics of playfulness that are inherent in their personalities. This is a fundamentally positive stance and represents a shared creative process geared towards enhancing well-being. As Magdalena Schamberger, the Artistic Director, comments:

> Trust and respect are the basis of all our work. Creating authentic connections and engagement with the individual are at its heart. Hope, laughter, and increased resilience are often a by-product. Our philosophy is to always look beyond the illness and ability of the person at their individual psychological and emotional needs,

thereby helping to overcome challenges such as stress, pain, frustration, loss of control and grief. (Personal communication)

Rachel Colles, one of the 'clowns', puts the relationship-building involved in the following terms:

I think what I like best is what I call 'the lucky secret' – an interaction between yourself, the person, and your partner; it's something the three of us have created, a moment of connection, which can be quite profound. (Personal communication)

Within this we can infer a connection between playful relationship-building and the nurturing of creativity in the person who has dementia; the clown-work is oriented around facilitating an open and divergent frame of thinking and relating, which contributes to a discovery that is positive and holds meaning, even if only in the moment. Rachel employs the term 'product' in a different sense from the way we might normally conceive of the artistic product. She says, 'The product is the connection and is unquantifiable; it is a truthful and positive affect' (Colles, 2014).

I visited an assessment ward in a hospital in Central Scotland on a day when Elderflowers were working. These were some of the things I observed:

In one small lounge a gentleman was sitting on his own. The Elderflowers introduced themselves as Bonnie and Handsome. 'Better if you were Bonnie and Clyde', he said. The three of them then fantasised as to how this might work out in the institution. 'We could always shoot ourselves out of the premises', he suggested. A reference to the ukelele carried by Handsome led to a discussion on guitars. The man showed himself to be knowledgeable on the subject, and gave them some advice on makes and models.

Then the conversation took a more lighthearted turn and landed on modes of dress. He commented unfavourably on their choice of clothes for the occasion. Bonnie adopted the role of the dominant partner. She flounced around the room. 'I'm Bonnie and I don't do ironing', she proclaimed. Handsome ruefully observed: 'I'm just Bonnie's bag-carrier.' (Killick and Schamberger, 2015)

After I had observed the Elderflowers visit the assessment ward, I returned to the hospital at a later date to see what kind of impact the session had made on the participants. The following is part of the account I wrote:

> I showed Vera a photograph of the two actors she had met with in the session a week previously. I reminded her of their names: 'Honey Bunch' and 'Sweetie Pie'.
>
> Then I produced a red nose from my pocket similar to the ones they had worn, and to the one she had been lent by them on that occasion. She took it from me and put it on. 'I think the noses are good', she said. Then, handing it back, she told me: 'Put it away. I wouldn't like it to be harmed. Till they come again.'
>
> She pointed to the photograph: 'They're beautiful children. They must be full of fun. They don't make me feel sad. I'm always very pleased to see them.'
>
> She went on to point to the male actor: 'Someone he loved very much might have died, so he's sad too in a way. They're definitely actors. I talk to them and they talk to me nicely. They play with me, chase me, and I pretend to run very fast. They make me laugh, but only as an act. I like to join in, in very small bits, correcting them. They are my friends, I like them very much.'
>
> Then she sang the whole of the Scottish song 'My Ain Folk' and commented: 'I see them as funny and sad and friendly.' (Killick, 2003)

2. HEATHER HILL AND DANCE

Dance is a very recent addition to the creative outlets offered to people with dementia. In Britain, its growth over the last decade has been remarkable, with an ever-increasing number of individual practitioners and organisations offering their assistance. In Australia,

Heather Hill has been the pioneer, presenting and writing widely on the subject. In her broad view of dance, she eschews the emphasis on technical expertise, instead asserting that dance is an activity open to all, irrespective of their subjective ability. Bodies are the focus, and she emphasises that we are all embodied beings. We have to get over the fear of making a display of ourselves and embrace the vision that expressive movement is an essential human activity. She employs every means available: spontaneous reactions, folk (and other types of dance), recorded music, props, nature, touch, singing and musical instruments. She sees physical handicap as no bar to participation and has worked with practically immobile persons: moving a wheelchair and certain movements while in a wheelchair are possibilities. She quotes a teacher who sees moving an eyebrow as a contribution!

Music is an important part of the work and it is crucial to choose it appropriately. It is not always about moving to a piece of music, which can be confining. Often it is a matter of starting from the kind of movement to be explored and then finding the right music to accompany it. Hill has spoken of her excitement when she has been able to work with a musician who has been able to improvise, and then a conversation between the two art-forms can develop. This provides the opportunity to respond in the moment, and capitalises on the creativity of dancer, musician and participant. In a remarkable article 'A Space to Be Myself' Hill (2003) sets out the parameters of a series of sessions with Elsie, where the development was rapid and rewarding (it formed part of a research study Hill was completing). Elsie was an 85-year-old lady with moderate dementia who had been admitted to a psychiatric hospital with a view to her being assessed for admission to an aged care facility. She had already taken part in some group sessions but otherwise Hill knew little about her. On these occasions an improvising musician was on hand.

Hill had four sessions, and all of them were videotaped, and viewed by Elsie and herself, which in turn were videotaped, giving the maximum information about verbal and non-verbal responses. Elsie's daughter also viewed the videos and commented on them. The study was therefore designed to obtain multiple perspectives, and through varying modalities. Amongst the significant findings were that in the first session focus, quality of movement and emotional involvement on Elsie's part steadily increased. Throughout the other sessions these qualities developed, as did the relationships between the three creative personalities involved. Elsie seemed to become more integrated, and her comments grew commensurately more coherent and apposite. Here are some examples:

> 'Thank you for bringing me out of my shell.'

> 'I've got together again.'

> 'It's brought the dullness out from me…to the brightness.'

> 'I think it's brought me out… Wake up.'

> 'So that's brought me out of my shell.'

Hill's conclusions are:

> I believe that dance offered Elsie a space and time to be herself – in dancing she could re-discover her 'old' self and re-experience it in the present. The viewing of the videos allowed her to reflect on the experience and reinforce it. The good feelings remained with her even after the sessions. For me, the enduring image of Elsie is one of a person in a state of ease with herself rather than of dis-ease and fragmentation. (Hill, 2003, p.39)

The principle Hill is describing here is what Kontos (2004, p.846) terms 'embodied selfhood'. She identifies 'the intrinsic corporeality of people's being-in-the-world'. In her research in care homes Kontos observed that '[t]he coherence of selfhood and its generative spontaneity persist despite the presence and progression of Alzheimer's because it resides below the level of cognition and in the pre-reflective level of experience (Kontos, 2004, p.845).

The idea that creativity resides at a level beyond cognition fits the idea of a creative process that is spontaneous and not tied to verbal conscious thinking. In this sense, creativity is a process that is linked with the expression of selfhood at a fundamental level and also relates to embodied ways of sense-making, knowing and relating.

3. IAN MCQUEEN AND POETRY

For over two decades I have been writing down the words of people with dementia and sometimes giving them back to them in the form of poetry. Mine is an editorial role, in which I have to decide what to leave out, but never put in any words of my own. A significant by-product of this affirming process is that in many instances I have been granted permission to publish these pieces. This has led to a number of books, the three earliest of these, sadly, anonymously as far as the authors were concerned, because of the sensitivities of care staff and relatives; the more recent ones with full credit to the individuals concerned. Those with whom I have collaborated have been at various stages of their dementia journey; the only section of the population to be thinly represented – out of necessity rather than choice – were those who, for whatever reasons, no longer employed verbal expression.

Some of the most striking poems have come from those in the early stage of the condition, as these tend to be the most articulate. These form a small but significant group, because they are likely to be the most active and forthright individuals. In 2003 the BBC approached me to make a programme about the process of making the poems, and I chose three people from this category to work with, one of whom was Ian McQueen.

At the time Ian was 59 and lived with his wife in a small town just outside Glasgow. He pronounced himself hostile to the idea of making poems, having had a bad school experience of the subject, but I persuaded him to let me record conversations with him in his home and leave it to me to decide on any poetic content that might result.

I paid him seven visits over a period of three months and recorded the whole evening's interactions on each occasion. Ian proved to be a remarkable subject: excited, voluble and highly imaginative in his ideas and use of language to express them.

I made a number of poems of transcribed speech, and each time I took them back to him he was astonished by, and rather proud of, the outcome. Ian was engaged in a struggle to remain cognitively intact and treated the sessions as occasions to 'get things off his chest'. He would often lose the thread of what he wanted to say, and on one occasion commented: 'Look, the little creature, it's running along the skirting-board and disappearing with my thought.'

In one of the poems in which Ian meets the challenge of memory-loss most positively, 'Taking Care of the Halo', the idea is that, just as in many religious paintings holy personages have halos round their heads, so in a secular context he invokes the halo to ward off the evil spirit of Alzheimer's:

> In there this old boy's saying, 'This is ok', or mebbe, 'We'll need to pull this back a wee bit.' It's like throw the rope out and pull it in, throw the rope out and pull it in. And you're doing that all the time; the brain's doing that all the time. It seems to be just patterns that come, do whatever they're doing, disappear, and then they probably come right round the back and do it again. Because my attitude is there's just like a halo or something like that round there, and it has to be there. Because that's the kingpin, that's the bit that sees up, down, over – all these things, and that's the thing you really have to take care of, otherwise you can get hurt very badly and very quickly.

By the end of the collaboration Ian had changed his mind about what poetry can do: 'A poem is something that feels into my psyche. It is where it comes out and where it ends up – essence of essences. What matters to me is the "me"-ness of it' (Killick, 2009).

The creation of poems by people with dementia, and by others from their words, is largely one necessarily confined to those for whom verbal language is still the preferred means of communication. Because of changes in the brain and the way it processes thought and turns it into speech, the language that comes out may differ from that employed in 'normal' discourse; there is some evidence, currently only anecdotal, that in many individuals it displays an effortless quality which comes from spontaneity unhindered by the censorship of the intellect. I call this 'the poetry of natural speech'. Peter Elbow terms it 'vernacular eloquence' (Elbow, 2012, p.7). A person with dementia said to me one day: 'I bet you've never been so near nature before.' I took this to mean that she was aware of becoming a person without disguises. This judgement can be applied to the nature of her utterances, too. In these instances there seems to be no barrier to hinder the expressive content from finding fresh creative outlets.

VALUING CREATIVITY

There is an argument about our society not valuing creativity enough. There is an even more powerful argument about not valuing the creativity of people with dementia sufficiently. The one, of course, feeds into the other. Creativity takes its place alongside other qualities displayed by people with dementia that are largely ignored: humour, insight and expressions of loving care.

Fundamentally, we don't value these attributes because we don't value people with dementia: we treat them as problems, inconveniences, even wastes of space, so we pour our limited resources into trying to find a cure so that dementia itself can be abolished; but the risk is this may well turn out to be like chasing a chimera.

In this context, even asking for creativity to be considered seems an impertinence. Nevertheless that is what we should do; it must take its place alongside a raft of other psycho-social initiatives to counter the negativity that threatens at all times to engulf those living with dementia.

We need a concerted effort to raise the profile of creativity, by means of talks, workshops, films and exhibitions, and especially by infiltrating popular media outlets such as newspapers, magazines, TV and radio programmes, and websites. It will be an uphill struggle, but as we have seen the examples of excellence are there – we just need to get the message across.

That involves consciousness-raising, but there also needs to be greater awareness through the institutions of society. People must be told at diagnosis that artistic stimulus can be a real component of future well-being. Doctors need to know what facilities exist in their area, and day centres should employ artists to supplement their more bread-and-butter provision. Care homes should invest in creativity as a part of their activities programmes. Arts venues should become dementia-friendly. Communities must be more supportive.

EVALUATING CREATIVITY

There is a sense in which it should be unnecessary for us to have to prove the importance of the role of the arts in the context of dementia – the examples should speak for themselves. This would be true of the works being produced and of the reactions of those taking part in the activities provided. Just bringing people into contact with people living with dementia seems to have a positive therapeutic effect: 'Actors (and artists) have a particular talent for communicating with people with dementia...[that] stems from a quality of attention, concentration, perhaps ability to be still "in the moment", filtering out all other distractions and claims on attention' (Benson, 2009, p.21).

With process becoming more accepted in the wider art-world as a legitimate source of study and appreciation, perhaps in the course of time a focus on this in relation to dementia may prove acceptable. In the meantime, funders and researchers still maintain an emphasis on traditional methods of evaluation. Basting points to fundamental drawbacks in this area:

> There are very few studies of the impact of the arts in caring for people with dementia of the scale and design that satisfy researchers used to pharmaceutical research designs. Studies of arts interventions are commonly excluded from systematic reviews because of weaknesses in study design such as the small number of people studied, poor descriptions of the intervention used. (Basting, 2014, p.135)

The basic problem is that responses are so individualised and intermittent, they do not lend themselves easily to statistical collection and analysis. A multi-targeted approach would seem to be the best option, which could consist of some or all of the following: interviews with participants; Dementia Care Mapping; questionnaires filled out by staff, relatives and some participants; journals kept by artists; videos, sound recordings and photographs of sessions (Basting and Killick, 2003).

A similar verdict has been reached over evaluating the effectiveness of art therapies for people with dementia. Beard (2012) critiqued the evidence base of music, visual arts, drama and dance over a 20-year period. His findings were depressing in terms of positive results. Although some studies recorded short-term gains in terms of engagement and mood, there was little evidence across studies of longer-lasting improvement in attention or sociability. There is a serious lack of longitudinal studies that might provide more convincing evidence of the efficacy of the approaches used. In addition, many of the studies were poorly designed and documented, there was no consensus over the measurement tools to be used, or whether to use process or product as core concepts. Critically, direct consultation with participants has been rare. Until researchers begin to remove the blinkers of the biomedical approach, it seems unlikely that we will have valuable evidence to present that will convince commissioners of services to invest in arts therapies. This is a case of anecdotal accounts far outstripping our current ability to register positive outcomes in research terms.

CONCLUSIONS

In this chapter we have seen how creativity in dementia deserves special consideration. Creative activities of all kinds are important sources of flow, connectedness, positive emotion, meaning and, hence, subjective and psychological well-being in the moment. The process of creativity in dementia arguably takes precedence over creative products, and people living with dementia need and deserve social environments that are flexible and inclusive enough to help them capitalise on the windows of creative expression they can enjoy. Fundamentally, creativity goes beyond verbal cognition and is a vital way for people to express and maintain an embodied sense of positive meaning and selfhood.

The whole subject of the arts in healthcare has recently moved up the national agenda in Britain (Mental Health Foundation, 2011) and the USA (National Endowment for the Arts, 2013). Lerman (n.d.), Founding Artistic Director of Dance Exchange, sums up the spirit of optimism well:

> Sometimes art achieves what therapy, medicine, or the best care of health professionals cannot. Sometimes art even achieves something that's beyond the best intentions of the artist. These moments can feel like little miracles when they happen, but they are usually instances of art functioning as it normally does: inspiring motivation, engaging parts of people's bodies or brains that they haven't been using, or allowing them to transcend their environments for a little while.

Creativity is here to stay in the lives of an increasing number of people with dementia, and will play an even more crucial role in the future as the numbers of people with the condition increase.

Some years ago a lady who had been engaging in an art activity one-to-one with me, turned and said, with great conviction in her voice: 'The arts are all there is. Give them us!'

We have taken the first steps towards making this a reality.

USEFUL WEBSITES

The Society for the Arts in Dementia Care: www.cecd-society.org

The Creative Dementia Arts Network: www.creativedementia.org

Arts for Health: www.artsforhealth.org

The Australian Centre for Arts and Health: www.artsandhealth.org.au

National Center for Creative Aging: www.creativeaging.org

Pictures to Share: www.picturestoshare.co.uk

TimeSlips: www.timeslips.org

Dementia Positive: www.dementiapositive.co.uk

REFERENCES

Allan, K. (2008) 'Positive psychology: Using strengths and experiencing flow.' *Journal of Dementia Care 16*(6), 24–26.

Arnheim, R. (1986) New Essays on the Psychology of Art. Berkeley, CA: University of California Press.

Barron, F.X. and Harrington, D.M. (1981) 'Creativity, intelligence and personality.' *Annual Review of Psychology 32*, 439–476.

Basting, A.D. (2014) 'The Arts in Dementia Care.' In M. Downs and B. Bowers (eds) *Excellence in Dementia Care: Research into Practice.* Maidenhead: McGraw Hill.

Basting, A.D. and Killick, J. (2003) *The Arts and Dementia Care: A Resource Guide.* Brooklyn: National Center for Creative Aging.

Beard, R.L. (2012) 'Art therapies and dementia care: A systematic review.' *Dementia 11*(5), 633–656.

Benson, S. (2009) 'Ladder to the moon: Interactive theatre in care settings.' *Journal of Dementia Care 17*, 20–23.

Csikszentmihalyi, M. (1998) 'Implications of a Systems Perspective for the Study of Creativity.' In R. J. Sternberg (ed.) *Handbook of Creativity.* Cambridge: Cambridge University Press. [AQ]

Dawson, A. and Baller, W. (1972) 'Relationship between creative activity and the health of elderly persons.' *The Journal of Psychology: Interdisciplinary and Applied 82*(1), 49–58.

Dormandy, T. (2000) *Old Masters: Great Artists in Old Age.* London: Hambledon and London.

Elbow, P. (2012) *Vernacular Eloquence: What Speech Can Bring to Writing.* New York, NY: Oxford University Press.

Fisher, K., Bradley, J. and Specht, D. (1999) 'Successful aging and creativity in later life.' *Journal of Aging Studies 13*(4), 457–472.

Forgeard, M.J.C., Jayawickreme, E., Kern, M.L. and Seligman, M.E.P. (2011) 'Doing the right thing: Measuring well-being for public policy.' *International Journal of Wellbeing 1*, 79–106.

Guilford, J. (1967) *The Nature of Human Intelligence.* New York, NY: McGraw-Hill.

Hill, H. (2003) 'A Space to Be Myself.' *Signpost 7*, 3.

Houston, A. (2009) 'Making Things More Real.' *Journal of Dementia Care 17*(6), 20–21.

Kaufman, J.C. and Sternberg, R.J. (2010) *The Cambridge Handbook of Creativity*. New York, NY: Cambridge University Press.

Killick, J. (2003) 'Funny and sad and friendly: A drama project in Scotland.' *Journal of Dementia Care 1*(1), 24–26.

Killick, J. (2009) 'Dementia and me-ness: The poetry of Ian McQueen.' *Writing in Education 47*, 44–47.

Killick, J. and Schamberger, M. (2015) 'Clowning and connecting: Elderflowers ten years on.' *Journal of Dementia Care 23*(1), 19–21.

Kontos, P. (2004) 'Ethnographic reflections on selfhood, embodiment and Alzheimer's disease.' *Ageing and Society 24*(6), 829–849.

Lindauer, M. (1992) 'Creativity in aging artists: Contributions from the humanities to the psychology of old age.' *Creativity Research Journal 5*(3), 211–231.

Lindauer, M.S. (1993) 'The old-age style and its artists.' *Empirical Studies and the Arts 11*, 135–146.

Lindauer, M. (2003) *Aging, Creativity and Art: A Positive Perspective on Late-Life Development*. New York, NY: Kluwer Academic Press.

Lerman, L. (n.d.) Quoted in Dance Exchange 'MetLife Foundation Healthy Living Initiative at Dance Exchange', available at http://danceexchange.org/projects/metlife-foundation-healthy-living-initiative, accessed on 10 June 2016.

Mental Health Foundation (2011) 'An Evidence Review of the Impact of Participatory Arts on Older People.' London: Mental Health Foundation.

Nachmanovitch, S. (1990) *Free Play: Improvisation in Life and Art*. New York, NY:Tarcher/Putnam.

Nakamura, J. and Czikszentmihalyi, M. (2005) 'The Concept of Flow.' In C.R. Snyder and S.J. Lopez (eds) *Handbook of Positive Psychology*. New York, NY: Oxford University Press.

National Endowment for the Arts (2013) *The Arts and Aging: Building the Science*. Washington, DC.

Peterson, C. and Seligman, M. (2004) *Character Strengths and Virtues: A Handbook and Classification*. New York, NY: Oxford University Press.

Searle, A. (2015) 'Genius at work – but you'll be lucky to catch the best bits.' *The Guardian*, 17 January 2015.

Sternberg, R. and Lubart, T. (1999) 'The Concept of Creativity.' In R. Sternberg (ed.) *Handbook of Creativity*. New York, NY: Cambridge University Press.

Takeuchi, H., Taki, Y., Sassa, Y., Hashizume, H. et al. (2010). 'White matter structures associated with creativity: Evidence from diffusion tensor imaging.' *NeuroImage 52*, 11–18.

Chapter 9

SPIRITUALITY AND WISDOM

Andrew Norris and Bob Woods

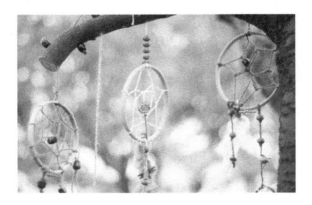

THE DISCOVERY OF THE PERSON WITH DEMENTIA

Advancing dementia challenges us with fundamental questions regarding what it means to be truly human. What defines our humanity and the essence of who we are? Do we merely 'exist' in a physical/ organic sense or what is it that gives meaning and purpose to our lives? It is here that exploring the concepts of spirituality and wisdom and how they apply to those living with dementia comes into play.

Despite similarities in the way people diagnosed with a particular type of dementia may present themselves, underneath it all, there still remains something that defines each person as an individual. This challenges an assumption often held in our society as a whole, let alone in the field of dementia, that people are defined and valued simply according to their cognitive abilities. Post (1995) described how a hyper-cognitive culture has developed, where those lacking the cognitive abilities required to function in our modern society with its plethora of pin numbers and passwords are deemed to be 'non-persons'.

A quarter of a century ago, one of us published a book for family caregivers, entitled *Alzheimer's Disease: Coping with a Living Death* (Woods, 1989). The sub-title was a direct quote from a family caregiver of a person with dementia and conveyed the sense of loss, grief and bereavement reported by many in this situation, before and since. Whilst this reflected the reality of the situation for that carer, describing dementia as a 'living death' places people living with dementia in the same conceptual category as the 'zombie' of popular culture. As Behuniak (2011) demonstrates, linking the experience of dementia with the image of zombies perpetuates hopelessness and stigma that may be attributed, at least in part, to our existential fear of losing cognitive abilities and of what is seen as a slow, distressing demise. The consequence is that people who are cognitively impaired can so easily be perceived as being less (or other) than human. For example, people with dementia and zombies are described with exceptional physical characteristics, such as shuffling, wandering, moaning; they may fail to recognise others, or indeed themselves. The use of the term 'victims' for people with dementia and caregivers suggests a condition that consumes (even 'cannibalises') living human beings and causes horror to those not yet afflicted; the emphasis on the increasing numbers to be affected across the world suggests an unstoppable plague of epidemic proportions. Finally, the zombie's all-pervading sense of hopelessness leads to death being seen as preferable to continued life in this condition. This preference for death over living with advanced dementia is mirrored in surveys of the general public's ratings of a variety of health states (Patrick *et al.*, 1994).

Tom Kitwood's contributions to our understanding of personhood, as we have seen in Chapter 2, take us towards a deep and rich understanding of what it means to be human, thus helping us reject the zombie metaphor. Kitwood (1997) encouraged us to take seriously the perspectives of people with dementia, to see the person behind the diagnostic label and therefore avoid dehumanising attitudes and practices. The many first-hand accounts now available contributed by people living with dementia make this much less of a challenge than say 20 years ago, when it was simply assumed that people with dementia could not make a meaningful contribution to understanding the experience of dementia (Woods, 1999; Woods 2001).

The challenge of advanced dementia remains, where cognitive impairment is so great that communication becomes difficult, and where the person requires support with the basic daily functions of life. Here, in his conceptualisation, Kitwood shows that personhood is still possible, in that it depends neither on cognition nor on the ability to take part in activities. Rather, at its heart is the relationship between the person with dementia and those around him or her who have the power to maintain personhood or detract from it.

SPIRITUALITY

There has been a considerable increase in interest over the past few decades in exploring how the concept of spirituality can be applied and is of relevance to addressing the needs of those living with dementia. This has partly been fuelled by insights expressed by a number of writers who themselves have been in the early stages of dementia (Bryden, 2005; Davis, 1993) but also reflects a growing recognition that those aspects of life that provide meaning and purpose, including religion, can have a significant impact on the well-being of people as they get older (Coleman and O'Hanlon, 2004). Walker (2013) reviewed a number of the ways in which positive spiritual well-being can lead to other positive factors in older people's lives, such as health and resilience. Coupled in particular with increasing frustration and impatience with the lack of progress towards finding a cure for dementia, growing consideration of spiritual well-being also highlights the importance of giving expression to the wisdom of the person living with dementia, accumulated through the experience of travelling a life-long journey.

So what is spirituality and how does it contribute towards our understanding and approach to supporting those living with dementia? In fact, spirituality has been notoriously difficult to define, partly because it deals with abstract concepts that are difficult to measure and partly because it has often been confused with and confined by its relationship to religious activity. Koenig, McCullough and Larson (2001, p.18) define spirituality thus:

> ...the personal quest for understanding answers to ultimate questions about life, about meaning and about relationship to the sacred or transcendent which may (or may not) lead to or arise from the development of religious rituals and the formation of community.

However, already we have here a suggestion that spirituality involves planned and deliberate acts that potentially involve cognitive purpose, which could be a challenge for a person living with advanced dementia. In an earlier definition, Patel, Naik and Humphries (1998, p.27) suggest that spirituality is 'the human search for personal meaning and mutually fulfilling relationships between people and the natural environment and between religious people and God'. Whilst this is more broadly encompassing, it still points to confusion with the expression of faith and religious belief. On the other hand, Mowat (2004) takes a broader view in suggesting that to age successfully, all of us are involved in a spiritual journey through which we discover meaning and find how we are located in the world. She suggests that this is vital if we are to achieve a sense of well-being and contentment as we grow older.

In a specific acknowledgment of how spirituality may apply to the world of the person living with dementia, MacKinlay (2001) describes spirituality in terms of that which enables the person to find meaning and hope. In her model of spiritual development, akin to Erikson's description of psycho-social growth, MacKinlay (2006, 2010) also goes on to suggest that a well-developed sense of spiritual well-being is likely to be associated with successfully resolving issues to do with vulnerability, isolation and fear, which older people are particularly likely to face. Echoing the thinking of Moody (1998), Walker (2013, p.156) proposes that 'self-determined wisdom; the discovery of meaning in ageing; an acceptance of the totality of life; revival of spirituality; preparation for death are all associated with spiritual well-being'.

One of the present authors, Norris (2013, p.207), proposed that 'embracing a person's spiritual needs is concerned with recognising how their story reflects what gives meaning and purpose in their life and helping to find ways in which that spirituality can be expressed'. He goes on to say that spiritual need is also related to a desire or yearning for development, growth and change. This approach to defining spirituality has far more practical implications and can lead to a better understanding of how attention to the spiritual dimension of a person's life can be achieved and the benefits that can be derived from doing so. In particular, Norris suggests that a useful way of understanding a person's spirituality is to examine their lives in terms of their past, present and future (see Figure 9.1).

How do people express their spirituality?

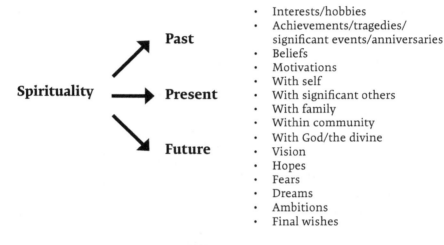

- Interests/hobbies
- Achievements/tragedies/ significant events/anniversaries
- Beliefs
- Motivations
- With self
- With significant others
- With family
- Within community
- With God/the divine
- Vision
- Hopes
- Fears
- Dreams
- Ambitions
- Final wishes

Figure 9.1: Expressions of spirituality

This perspective suggests that present and future spirituality build on and link with past experiences, beliefs and values. In the context of dementia, autobiographical memory, which makes a major contribution to our sense of identity, may have an important role to play in relation to spirituality. Autobiographical memory does not appear in general to function akin to a video recording of our lives but involves reconstructive processes, which are influenced by our emotions and by the way we wish to present ourselves. Although memories for the earlier parts of life are typically thought to be relatively spared in early stages of dementia at least, there can be some impairment, when put to the test. As autobiographical memories are generally least well recalled from the middle stages of life, there is a risk of a disconnection in autobiographical memory, with the person with dementia recalling memories from their early years, but not being able to make the connection with their current situation and circumstances.

The popularity of reminiscence approaches over the years may be attributable to the connections made through triggering and prompting memories of past experiences and events, in a group context or on an individual basis. Life review – a therapeutic approach initially developed by Butler (1963) – involves the person working through their life story, typically chronologically, reflecting on and evaluating their experiences. In Erikson's (1963) theory of life-span development, this type of life review process is seen as underpinning the developmental task of later life. The poles of this task reflect at the one extreme, a sense of integrity, a life well-lived, with failures and disappointments seen in the context of achievements and satisfaction; at the other extreme is despair, where regrets, resentment and sadness outweigh any positive considerations.

In studies with people with dementia, an approach derived from Butler's life review therapy, used individually to develop a life-story book, has been shown to improve autobiographical memory, as well as leading to benefits in aspects of well-being (Morgan and Woods, 2010; Subramaniam, Woods and Whitaker, 2014). This suggests that it is feasible to support the contribution of the past to current and future spirituality in people living with dementia. The past does not, of course, necessarily determine the present or future, and people with dementia, as the rest of us, should have the opportunity to make new choices, develop new preferences, abandon previous habits and develop new insights, even if these changes appear inconsistent with what was seen as the person's core self (Woods and Pratt, 2005).

The model proposed by Norris in this chapter points to the importance of current relationships as being a vehicle for feeding and expressing an individual's spiritual well-being. It also indicates that, whilst being an important component of the way in which spirituality is expressed in the present moment through a relationship with the divine, this is by no means the only way by which this can be achieved. Within what is often a context of pessimism and hopelessness in relation to the progressively deteriorating nature of dementia, this model also highlights the importance of keeping a sense of hope and the future alive. Even if later life cannot be enjoyed in the way once envisaged, this does not invalidate the need or the possibility that expressed desires or hopes, which have been extrapolated from previous indications of preference or projection, cannot be addressed and realised.

There will also be anxieties about the end of life, however explicitly expressed, and it is important that space and opportunity for these to be explored is given. Even if a person is not able to articulate their concerns, it is vital to provide a sensitive and supportive environment where comfort and reassurance are available. Kitwood highlighted 'hope' as a key feature of well-being in dementia, and this may be interpreted as a sense that 'all will be well', even in the midst of uncertainty and confusion. The person with dementia who has this sense of hope perceives that those around him or her are supportive rather than threatening, that he or she is known and valued as an individual and that he or she will not come to harm.

Given that tapping into and providing opportunities for expression of the spiritual dimension to people's lives is important, especially when conceptualised in this broadest sense, the question remains as to how this can be achieved with those living with dementia, for whom opportunity and choice will be much more restricted. We will return to this topic having first considered the links between spirituality, wisdom and creative expression.

WISDOM

It is often considered that there may be a relationship between spirituality and wisdom. From the perspective of the model shown earlier, this might, for example, be based on the accumulated experience of one's past. Wisdom is certainly just as challenging to define as is spirituality! Wisdom has been described as a hidden treasure of old age (Baltes, Dittmann-Kohli and Dixon, 1984) and is perhaps one of the few characteristics for which people expect a positive trajectory in later life (Heckhausen, Dixon and Baltes, 1999). Wisdom is described as both a predictor and product of successful ageing, with numerous cross-sectional studies suggesting that it is more robustly linked to well-being than physical health, socio-economic status and the physical environment (see Peterson and Seligman, 2004).

Does this imply that living a long time makes a person wise? Just as important may be the ability to reflect on experience, to see the 'bigger picture' of actions in their context, and to drill down to the essence of life and relationship. Baltes and Kunzmann (2003, p.131) provide an operational definition of wisdom as 'expert knowledge and judgement about important, difficult and uncertain questions associated with the meaning and conduct of life'. This definition relates to the essence of the human condition and the ways and means of planning, managing and understanding a good life.

In these terms, dementia might, at first sight, seem a barrier to wisdom, or at least to the expression of it. Expert knowledge may have been accumulated, but is the exercise of judgement possible as cognitive impairment develops? Just as it is unlikely that all older people have a high degree of wisdom, perhaps the same may be the case for people with dementia. Those who are (understandably perhaps) preoccupied with their own concerns and anxieties may not find the opportunity to reflect on what lies behind the actions and words of those around them. But those who work in dementia care may well have witnessed moments when the person with dementia 'hits the nail on the head', with a remark or an action that cuts through day-to-day busy-ness and the defences we use to present an image to the world: perhaps recognising and validating the feelings of someone around them – a relative, a care worker, another person with dementia – reaching, in the moment, the essence of an emotion or a relationship that has evaded those who are purportedly 'cognitively intact'. In these moments of wisdom, the person with dementia is not concerned with badges of status and authority; they may not show due deference or wrap up raw emotions in the web of culturally accepted language; and instead of beating about the bush, they may reach inside the core of human existence.

Perhaps this type of wisdom comes closer to Erikson's (1982) definition of wisdom as a kind of 'informed and detached concern with life itself in the face of death itself' (p.61). The role of wisdom is seen as being 'to guide our investment in sight and sound and to focus our capacities on what is relevant, enduring and nourishing, both for us individually and for the society in which we live' (Erikson, 1998, p.7). The person with dementia may no longer be an active participant in many of the diversionary activities and pursuits that have developed to fill the time between birth and death, and may thus be free from the cultural restrictions and expectations that govern politeness and etiquette. However, the person may remain a human observer of the merry-go-round of life and his or her observations may have a depth that goes beyond the sophisticated, nuanced explanations of those who have not yet been able to break free.

Joan Erikson developed her husband's work on later life following his death. When asked, 'What is real wisdom?' she replied that it 'comes from life experience, well digested. It's not what comes from reading great books. When it comes to understanding life, experiential learning is the only worthwhile kind; everything else is hearsay' (Goleman, 1988).

People with dementia may surprise us by the way in which their life-time of experiential learning at times shines an unexpected light on our understanding of life.

CREATIVE EXPRESSION

Creative arts programmes have become very popular in the context of dementia care (these are discussed in more depth in Chapter 8). They appear to offer a potential route to aesthetic appreciation and expression and to break free from a world where cognition dominates. Creative arts offer an experience that could equally involve the emotions and spirit, the appreciation of beauty and of cultural themes, and the opportunity for self-expression in ways that may circumvent difficulties with language and memory. Such programmes take a number of forms. The arts engagement programme at New York's Museum of Modern Art (MoMA) was a pioneering project, but there are examples of participation in choirs, art classes, dance groups, theatre and drama, creative writing activities, galleries and exhibitions from across the UK and many other countries. In the UK, the Alzheimer's Society 'Singing for the Brain' programme offers people with dementia and carers the opportunity to sing together in the context of a choir, and it has long been known that listening to preferred music can result in a positive response from many people with dementia.

There are many anecdotal reports of benefits from these sorts of programmes, but generally it has proved more difficult to pin down the exact benefits in more rigorous evaluations. Typically, people with dementia become more engaged during the creative activity itself (MacPherson et al., 2009; Salisbury, Algar and Windle, 2011). Camic, Tischler and Pearman (2014) report an evaluation of a 'Viewing and making art together' programme. This was an eight-week art gallery-based intervention offered at two distinctly different galleries for 12 people with mild to moderate dementia and their carers. The researchers reported: 'Participants were unanimous in their enjoyment and satisfaction with the programme, despite the lack of significance from standardised measures.' Camic, Baker and Tischler (2015) present a model of how the intervention has an effect on people with dementia and carers, based on qualitative interviews with participants. The gallery is seen as a 'special and valued place', with the art providing intellectual stimulation and engagement, and promoting positive emotions and social interaction and connections. Similarly, Flatt and colleagues (2015) describe cognitive stimulation and self-esteem arising from a similar programme in the USA. People living with dementia described feeling accepted and valued, with the art both connecting with their personal experience and enabling a shared experience with the other participants.

The growing body of research in this area certainly supports the view that dementia does not inevitably take away the potential for aesthetic appreciation, although as MacPherson et al. (2009) suggest, this may be 'for the moment'. Such moments of connection, engagement, emotion and expression fit well with a broader concept of spirituality. The ability of these programmes to change the perceptions of others regarding dementia (Camic et al., 2015) may also be especially important in allowing people living with dementia to have the opportunity for creative expression and a form of spiritual experience. There are of course a range of activities that might be enjoyed by significant numbers of people with dementia, but because artistic and cultural activities are typically valued in society, participation in these preferentially challenges the stigma of dementia. Especially when there are discernible *outputs* (e.g. a performance by a choir of people with dementia as part of a concert or an exhibition of artwork by people with dementia in a gallery), the potential contribution to society of people with dementia becomes even more apparent. People are then transformed from simply being the recipients of care, to having a role to play that is meaningful and valued. This is essential if people living with dementia are to be real partners in 'dementia-friendly communities'. Only then will the fear so often associated with public attitudes to dementia be replaced by a fuller appreciation of the complex, multi-faceted nature of the experience of dementia.

RELIGION

Thus far we have not referred in any detail to the one aspect of living that is often most associated with the spiritual dimension of life – namely religion. This has been deliberate, to emphasise the point that spirituality is broader than religion. However, religion can be an extremely important channel for expressing spirituality. As Coleman and O'Hanlon (2004) suggest, spirituality is usually associated with a belief in some kind of transcendent or supernatural force. As with our model of spirituality, the importance of religious belief can also be couched in terms of how it relates to the past, present and future, not least for those living with dementia.

The availability and familiarity of a vast resource of religious writing, scriptures, hymnody and prayers can provide significant comfort for many, sometimes including those without a formal faith background. At the very least, they provide a gateway to a real depth of being, often untouched by other human experiences. Coupled with this is the way that religious ritual, as with many familiar routines, can provide a vehicle for making sense of an otherwise chaotic world that people, and especially those living with dementia, face. This has led to an increased focus on how acts of worship and sacred environments can be made more 'dementia-friendly' by paying attention to such characteristics as the importance of familiarity, creating the right ambience, use of multisensory approaches, etc. (Kennedy *et al.*, 2014). There are also an increasing number of resources available to help worship leaders to plan worship themes suitable for those living with dementia (Scripture Union, 2010).

These trends place importance on being able to engage with people in the here and now and to facilitate opportunities to engage with the transcendent. From a psycho-social perspective, the early writings of Erikson (1963), later taken up Tornstam (1994, 1999) and developed by Joan Erikson (1998), recognised the importance of the place of the transcendent using the concept of 'gerotranscendance', to describe those who reach a state of peaceful acceptance, overcoming fear of death, as they near the end of their lives.

With regard to hopes for the future and beyond this life, of course religious belief and faith have much to offer the believer. And there are many examples too, of those who have found faith on their death-bed as they are confronted with their finitude. Whilst not an excuse for proselytising, ministry at the end of life can offer great hope and support to both those whose end is near and those who care for them.

THE EFFECTS OF DEMENTIA ON SPIRITUALITY

Here we consider first-hand accounts of how dementia has affected a pre-existing faith or spiritual life. Jim McWade is a retired Methodist minister, living with his wife in North Wales, who has talked about his dementia on TV and radio and in an interview with the Alzheimer's Society magazine *Living with Dementia* (February, 2009). He describes the diagnosis coming as a 'big bang', a sudden complete upheaval of his life. He reports feelings of sadness and loss, becoming emotional and taking some time to come to terms with the situation so that he could face it: 'The focus had shifted from God to a whole new problematic world of Alzheimer's and doctors. I was preoccupied with doubt and worry and felt as though I was on an island with not another soul around' (p.6).

However, after about six months he felt God 'knocking at the door again', wanting to be let back in, and Jim's spiritual life was renewed. Jim describes his ultimate fear as being so impaired he is unable to 'wonder at God'; he is content to relinquish his clerical collar and not to be responsible for solving major problems as long as he is able to feel that 'this mortal frame of mine is part of the loving and caring God' (pp.6–7).

Insights from qualitative interviews with a further six people with mild to moderate dementia who had a pre-existing religious or spiritual life are analysed by Dalby, Sperlinger and Boddington (2011). The participants similarly described an essential continuity of their spiritual experience, of their relationship with a divine being, and an acceptance of death to come. A search for meaning in the experience of dementia was reported. Some asked 'Why me?' whilst others viewed dementia as a spiritual challenge and saw themselves as now having greater compassion for others. Despite the sense of continuity, participants recognised that they had changed and were experiencing losses. This meant they could not now always express their spirituality as they had previously. To an extent, there was a sense in which inside they might be the same person, but externally they could no longer function as they used to. Participants sought to find ways of coping with the changes experienced, and several described keeping hopeful in the face of dementia. Past memories and supportive family and friends were also helpful in maintaining a sense of self. All participants sought to sustain spiritual connection and expression, through holding onto their spiritual values and positive attitudes. Continuing with established spiritual practices, such as prayer, meditation or bible reading, and continuing to be part of a spiritual community were important. The person's relationships with others were essential for spiritual expression and connection. From a questionnaire study including 20 people with dementia recruited from a Memory Clinic, Jolley and colleagues (2010) also found that participants reported gaining comfort from spiritual practices associated with their beliefs, and there was no indication that the strength of their beliefs had lessened.

FROM TRIVIAL TO SPIRITUAL

The importance of the spiritual dimension in all our lives cannot be underestimated. However, it is evident that growing older brings with it particular issues that have to be faced and where a call on spiritual resources can be of great value. As Walker (2013) reminds us, it was the renowned psychotherapist Carl Jung (1960) who suggested that later life not only brings with it superior possibilities but actually constitutes what gives life its true purpose and meaning.

Much of what has been referred to in this chapter applies to everyone but is of special importance for those living with dementia. Snyder (2003) quotes a number of people living with dementia who provide insights into the importance of addressing spiritual issues when faced with their limitations:

> Having Alzheimer's disease made me face ultimate realities, not my bank account. My money, my job, and other parts of my life were trivial issues that restricted my growth, my spiritual growth. Alzheimer's disease transferred me from what I call the trivial plane to the spiritual or personal plane. I had to face the absolute horror of the 'A' word, and I began a dialogue with my existence, a dialogue with my life and my death. (p.299)

The powerful writings of Christine Bryden (2005), herself living with dementia, testify to the role that spirituality can play. She says, 'As cognition fades, spirituality can flourish as a source of identity' (see Mackinlay, 2002, p.71).

Not only would it seem that recognising and facilitating the opportunities for a person's spiritual being to have expression can positively affect their well-being, but the nature and experience of dementia also has something to teach us about what it means to be human. Goldsmith (1999) reminds us that whoever and whatever we are, from a Christian theological perspective, we are unconditionally accepted by God and this must be a great source of comfort and hope for those who live with this condition. However, more than this, as some have argued, free from the constraints and mores of social living, dementia can provide us with a more perfect way of being human (Saunders, 2002). There is always a danger in infantilising, but there are positive parallels to be drawn when considering such qualities as openness, trust and faith, which are manifested to some considerable degree in both. As Goodall (2013) reflects, 'The spiritual tasks of old age are not changed by dementia they are just made more difficult to see' (p.181). There is no doubt that to ignore them and to deny those living with dementia the opportunity to avail themselves of the depth of resource the spiritual dimension to life has to offer will seriously impoverish their well-being.

We conclude by returning to the fundamentals of what it means to be a person. Kitwood defined personhood as 'a standing or status that is bestowed upon one human being, by others, in the context of relationship and social being' (Kitwood, 1997, p.8). In this context we see that retaining spirituality ultimately may depend on those around the person with dementia remaining alongside the person as the journey progresses, holding onto the person's identity and life-story. Kitwood, a former Anglican priest, entertains the potential for spirituality in describing person-centred care in advanced dementia, citing the work of the Austrian-born theologian Martin Buber:

> In dementia many aspects of the psyche that had, for a long time, been individual and 'internal', are again made over to the interpersonal milieu...if there is a spirituality, it will most likely be of the kind that Buber describes, where the divine is encountered in the depth of I–thou relating. (Kitwood, 1997, p.69)

The challenge for those of us supporting and caring for people with dementia is to be able ourselves to be fully human in the interaction and the relationship, with all that entails. Experience suggests that it is only too easy for the person with dementia to be treated as less than human, to be objectified or infantilised. Relating in these terms may be characterised as 'I–it' rather than the very personal meeting of souls suggested by 'I–thou'.

Spirituality in dementia is not simply a challenge for the person living with a dementia: it is for those who provide support and care to find their own path to spirituality that allows them to be with people with dementia in a way that is fully human – a demanding, sometimes draining, but ultimately rewarding and enriching endeavour.

REFERENCES

Baltes, P.B., Dittmann-Kohli, F. and Dixon, R.A. (1984) 'New Perspectives on the Development of Intelligence in Adulthood: Toward a Dual-process Conception and a Model of Selective Optimization with Compensation.' In C. Snyder and S. Lopez (eds) *Handbook of Positive Psychology.* New York, NY: Oxford University Press.

Baltes, P.B. and Kunzmann, U. (2003) 'Wisdom.' *Psychologist 16*(3), 131–133.

Behuniak, S.M. (2011) 'The living dead? The construction of people with Alzheimer's disease as zombies.' *Ageing and Society 31*(1), 70.

Bryden, C. (2005) *Dancing with Dementia: My Story of Living Positively with Dementia.* London: Jessica Kingsley Publishers.

Butler, R.N. (1963) 'The life review: An interpretation of reminiscence in the aged.' *Psychiatry 26*, 65–76.

Camic, P.M., Baker, E.L. and Tischler, V. (2015) 'Theorizing how art gallery interventions impact people with dementia and their caregivers.' *The Gerontologist.* DOI: 10.1093/geront/gnv063

Camic, P.M., Tischler, V. and Pearman, C.H. (2014) 'Viewing and making art together: A multi-session art-gallery-based intervention for people with dementia and their carers.' *Aging and Mental Health 18*(2), 161–168.

Coleman, P.G. and O'Hanlon, A. (2004) *Ageing and Development.* London: Arnold/ Hodder.

Dalby, P., Sperlinger, D.J. and Boddington, S. (2011) 'The lived experience of spirituality and dementia in older people living with mild to moderate dementia.' *Dementia.* DOI: 10.1177/1471301211416608

Davis, R. (1993) *My Journey into Alzheimer's Disease: Helpful Insights for Family and Friends.* Amsterdam: Scripture Press.

Erikson, E. (1963) *Childhood and Society* (revised edn). New York, NY: W.W. Norton.

Erikson, E.H. (1982) *The Life Cycle Completed.* New York, NY: W.W. Norton.

Erikson, E.H. (1998) *The Life Cycle Completed* (extended version with new chapters on the ninth stage by Joan M. Erikson). New York, NY: W.W. Norton.

Flatt, J.D., Liptak, A., Oakley, M.A., Gogan, J., Varner, T. and Lingler, J.H. (2015) 'Subjective experiences of an art museum engagement activity for persons with early-stage Alzheimer's disease and their family caregivers.' *American Journal of Alzheimer's Disease and Other Dementias.* DOI: 10.1177/1533317514549953

Goldsmith, M. (1999) 'Dementia: A Challenge to Christian Theology and Pastoral Care.' In A. Jewell (ed.) *Spirituality and Ageing.* London: Jessica Kingsley Publishers.

Goleman, D. (1988) 'Erikson, in his own old age, expands his view of life.' *New York Times* (14 June 1988). Available at www.nytimes.com/books/99/08/22/specials/erikson-old.html, accessed on 21 April 2016.

Goodall, M. (2013) 'Remember the Lord Your God!' In K. Albans and M. Johnson (eds) *God, Me and Being Very Old.* London: SCM Press.

Heckhausen, J., Dixon, R. and Baltes, P. (1999) 'Gains and losses in development throughout adulthood as perceived by different adult age groups.' *Developmental Psychology 25*, 109–121.

Jolley, D., Benbow, S.M., Grizzell, M., Willmott, S., Bawn, S. and Kingston, P. (2010) 'Spirituality and faith in dementia.' *Dementia 9*, 311–325.

Jung, C.G. (1960) 'The Stages of Life.' In *The Structure and Dynamics of the Psyche* (collected works of C.G. Jung, vol. 8). Princeton, NJ: Princeton University Press.

Kennedy, E., Allen, B., Hope, A. and James, I.A. (2014) 'Christian worship leaders' attitudes and observations of people with dementia.' *Dementia.* DOI: 10.1177/1471301213479786

Kitwood, T. (1997) *Dementia Reconsidered: The Person Comes First.* Buckingham: Open University Press.

Koenig, H.G., McCullough, M.E. and Larson, D.B. (2001) *Handbook of Religion and Health.* New York, NY: Oxford University Press.

MacKinlay, E. (2001) *The Spiritual Dimension of Ageing.* London: Jessica Kingsley Publishers.

MacKinlay, E. (2002) *Mental Health and Spirituality in Later Life.* Binghamton, NY: The Haworth Pastoral Press.

MacKinlay, E. (2006) *Spiritual Growth and Care in the Fourth Age.* London: Jessica Kingsley Publishers.

MacKinlay, E. (ed.) (2010) *Ageing and Spirituality Across Faiths and Cultures.* London: Jessica Kingsley Publishers.

MacPherson, S., Bird, M., Anderson, K., Davis, T. and Blair, A. (2009) 'An art gallery access programme for people with dementia: "You do it for the moment."' *Aging and Mental Health 13*(5), 744–752.

McWade, J. (2009) 'Keeping the Faith.' *Living with Dementia*, February 2009.

Moody, H. (1998) 'Does Old Age have Meaning?' In *Aging: Concepts and Controversies.* Thousand Oaks, CA: SAGE Publications.

Morgan, S. and Woods, R.T. (2010) 'Life review with people with dementia in care homes: A preliminary randomized controlled trial.' *Non-pharmacological Therapies in Dementia 1*, 43–60.

Mowat, H. (2004) 'Successful Ageing: The Spiritual Journey.' In A. Jewell (ed.) *Ageing, Spirituality and Well-being*. London: Jessica Kingsley Publishers.

Norris, A. (2013) 'Chaplaincy among Older People.' In K. Albans and M. Johnson (eds) *God, Me and Being Very Old*. London: SCM Press.

Patel, N., Naik, D. and Humphries, B. (1998) *Visions of Reality: Religion and Ethnicity in Social Work*. London: CCETSW.

Patrick, D.L., Starks, H.E., Cain, K.C., Uhlmann, R.F. and Pearlman, R.A. (1994) 'Measuring preferences for health states worse than death.' *Medical Decision Making 14*(1), 9–18.

Peterson, C. and Seligman, M. (2004) *Character Strengths and Virtues: A Handbook and Classification*. New York, NY: Oxford University Press.

Post, S.G. (1995) *The Moral Challenge of Alzheimer's Disease*. Baltimore, MD: John Hopkins University Press.

Salisbury, K., Algar, K. and Windle, G. (2011) 'Arts programmes and quality of life for people with dementia: A review.' *Journal of Dementia Care 19*(3), 33–37.

Saunders, J. (2002) *Dementia: Pastoral Theology and Pastoral Care*. Cambridge: Grove Books.

Scripture Union (2010) *Being with God* (a series of three booklets – *Words of Hope/Faith/Peace* – each containing 31 devotional outlines for individual or small group worship and CD of suggested hymns). Available at www.scriptureunion.org.uk/Shop/Biblereadingguides/Biblereadingforadults/BeingwithGod-fordementiasufferers/164915.id, accessed on 21 April 2016.

Snyder, L. (2003) 'Satisfactions and challenges in spiritual faith and practice for persons with dementia.' *Dementia 2*(3), 299–313.

Subramaniam, P., Woods, B. and Whitaker, C. (2014) 'Life review and life story books for people with mild to moderate dementia: A randomised controlled trial.' *Aging and Mental Health 18*, 363–375.

Tornstam, L. (1994) 'Gerotranscendence – A Theoretical and Empirical Exploration.' In L.E. Thomas and S.A. Eisenhandler (eds) *Aging and the Religious Dimension*. Westport, CT: Auburn.

Tornstam, L. (1999) 'Late-life Transcendence: A New Developmental Perspective on Aging.' In L.E. Thomas and S.A. Eisenhandler (eds) *Religion, Belief and Spirituality in Late Life*. New York, NY: Springer Publishing Co., Inc.

Walker, J. (2013) 'Long Life Discipleship in 2013 People.' In K. Albans and M. Johnson (eds) *God, Me and Being Very Old*. London: SCM Press.

Woods, B. (1999) 'The person in dementia care.' *Generations 23*(3), 35–39.

Woods, B. and Pratt, R. (2005) 'Awareness in dementia: Ethical and legal issues in relation to people with dementia.' *Aging and Mental Health 9*, 423–429.

Woods, R.T. (1989) *Alzheimer's Disease: Coping with a Living Death*. London: Souvenir Press.

Woods, R.T. (2001) 'Discovering the person with Alzheimer's disease: Cognitive, emotional and behavioural aspects.' *Aging and Mental Health 5*(1), S7–S16.

Chapter 10

POSITIVE PSYCHOLOGY AND RELATIONAL DEMENTIA CARE

CREATING AN 'ENRICHED ENVIRONMENT'

Tony Ryan and Mike Nolan

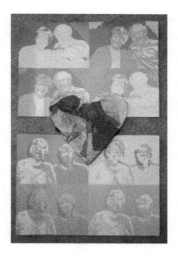

Kitwood's work...has rightly been considered to have altered the way that both dementia itself and the provision of care services are conceptualised today.

Baldwin and Capstick (2007)

INTRODUCTION

For us, this quote from a reader and critical commentary on the seminal contribution of Professor Tom Kitwood to the field of dementia care sets the scene for the arguments we will advance in this chapter on the central importance of relationships to any understanding of a positive psychology of dementia. Building on arguments relating to concepts such as 'successful ageing', we intend to be somewhat critical of the unchallenged acceptance of positivity (whilst retaining most of its precepts) in order to avoid what Held (2002) termed the 'tyranny of the positive attitude'. The quote rightly asserts Kitwood's influence on current thinking in dementia care but, as with positive psychology, we do not adopt his arguments uncritically and build on earlier calls for a more inclusive vision of dementia care research and practice (Nolan *et al.*, 2002) that is true to the principles of a relational model.

The chapter begins with a brief overview of debates relating to a positive psychology of ageing in general, particularly for people with what are now termed 'high support needs' (Katz *et al.*, 2011). It then moves on to consider what might loosely be termed 'a positive psychology of dementia', with a focus on the notion of personhood, before summarising current thinking on positive relationships for people with dementia. However, we intend to move well beyond this and argue that a relational view of dementia cannot focus on the needs of any one individual or group of individuals but rather must address the needs of all those involved in supporting people with dementia, whether in an unpaid or paid capacity. In so doing, we will outline a series of values that we believe should inform such an approach and that we think should be applied at multiple levels, ranging from the intrapersonal, through the interpersonal and community, to society as a whole. We will outline a framework, the 'Senses Framework' (Nolan *et al.*, 2006) and consider how it might be used to create an 'enriched environment' (Nolan *et al.*, 2006) that facilitates positive relationships in dementia care in a diversity of settings.

We deliberately draw primarily on the literature relating to ageing in general and older people living with dementia. This in no way seeks to deny or ignore the needs of younger people with dementia, for whom a positive and relational approach is as at least as important (Roach *et al.*, 2014). Rather, it recognises both that our understanding of the experiences of younger people with dementia and their families is currently limited (Roach *et al.*, 2014) and that to attempt to consider the needs of both older and younger people living with dementia, in a relatively brief chapter, would do justice to neither.

POSITIVE PSYCHOLOGY, RELATIONSHIPS AND AGEING

There is no universally accepted approach to understanding the experience of ageing, but recent trends have seen a move away from the search for 'grand' theories, which seek to provide a universal explanation of the ageing experience, towards models that adopt a more individualised approach in which personally constructed meanings created within social relationships figure far more prominently. Some of the earlier theories of ageing, such as activity theory (Havighurst, 1963) and selective optimisation (Baltes and Baltes, 1990), are primarily focused around function and its potential loss, with the notion of relationships being peripheral. Classical sociological theories of ageing have emerged from distinct positions within the discipline, such as functionalism (Cumming and Henry, 1961) and Marxist/political economy (Walker, 1981), which do not address the fundamental role of positive relationships but rather see ageing as being structurally imposed, principally through retirement and related policies. Life-course theories, such as socio-emotional selectivity theory, do address relationships, however, via a life-long continuum, suggesting that people's social needs change with age and that this is a developmental process, rather than socially imposed (Carstenson, Isaacowitz and Charles, 1999). Within socio-emotional selectivity theory, social networks are determined by age, with an expectation that these will reduce in later life. This reduction, it is argued, is as a response to the emotional needs of ageing, resulting in a 'pro-active pruning' towards a smaller number of close, intimate relationships (Carstenson et al., 1999, p.174). This need for positive relationships emerges again and more clearly in theories such as Gerotranscendence (Tornstam, 2005), which sees ageing as a transformational period of one's life during which well-being is positively achieved. Relationships within Tornstam's theory also undergo a process of reduction, with a focus on a smaller number of close positive relationships or even a single partner with whom to share thoughts and feelings. Tornstam (2005) claims that this solitude is often misinterpreted by younger people, who fail to recognise the significance of quiet contemplation. More generally, authors such as

Lang (2001) have highlighted both the importance of relationships to older people and the effort required to acquire, maintain, transform or discontinue such relationships. However, such arguments focus largely on motivational and cognitive processes (Lang, 2001), which, by definition, are challenged in dementia. We intend to argue that, despite this, relationships remain of central importance to people who have dementia and all those they engage with.

The above accounts are consistent with a 'grand' theory model of ageing. More clearly linked to the idea of seeing ageing as a positive experience are concepts such as 'successful ageing' (Rowe and Kahn, 1987), and the more recent, and politically driven, vision of 'active ageing' (World Health Organization, 2002). Whilst superficially positive, such approaches have come in for considerable criticism (Scheidt, Humphreys and Yorgason, 1999) from those who argue that they are elitist and ageist, casting those older people who do not live up to the definition of 'success' (usually revolving around high levels of physical and cognitive functioning) into the 'unsuccessful' category (Minkler, 1996). Building on the writings of Held (2002, 2004) this chimes with Aspinwall and Tedeschi's (2010) cautionary note about the dangers of accepting a positive approach uncritically. What is required, as Held (2004) argues of positive psychology in general, is a more 'nuanced' recognition that both negative and positive experiences are part of life. Following these tenets, we hope to provide a positive but realistic appreciation of the benefits of applying a relational model to dementia care so as to enhance the experiences of all parties.

Retaining a 'positive' emphasis, but also recognising the challenges that ageing imposes, more recent theoretical and empirical work has focused on understanding what creates a meaningful life for people with 'high support needs' (Katz et al., 2011), which would of course include people living with dementia. Building on a raft of work conducted over many years, the Joseph Rowntree Foundation have identified seven key challenges to improving the well-being of people with high support needs (Blood, 2013). The importance of relationships figures prominently as a key challenge: 'We must ensure that all support is founded in, and reflects, meaningful relationships. Connecting with others is a fundamental human need, whatever our age or support needs' (Blood, 2013, p.13).

The work of Katz and colleagues (2011) and others (e.g. Tanner, 2010; Roberts, 2012) credits older people, even those with high support needs, with having agency and actively 'managing' their lives to maintain optimum well-being. This provides clear points of connection, with models explicitly promoting a positive psychology of ageing (e.g. see Ranzijn, 2002a, 2000b) that highlight the importance of viewing older people not as passive recipients in need of care but as actively contributing, both to their own well-being and that of the wider social networks of which they are part. This shifts the focus to the relationships that older people have both with other people and their wider environment. Key concepts, such as resilience, are now emerging, which span both the literature on ageing in particular and on positive psychology more generally (Blane *et al.*, 2011; Janssen, Van Regenmortel and Abma, 2011). Within this literature it is social relationships and connections with community, rather than physical/mental functioning or socio-economic status, that capture the interactional and contextual nature of ageing. What is evident here is the need to adopt a broadly defined view of relationships that goes beyond the interpersonal domain and includes both wider social relationships, and also the relationships that older people have with the communities in which they live and the wider society of which they are part. It is this view of relationships that we adopt here and will now go on to consider as it relates to living positively with dementia.

POSITIVE PSYCHOLOGY, RELATIONSHIPS AND DEMENTIA

Chapter 2 has outlined the significance of the work of Tom Kitwood and, in particular, the notion of personhood, which is widely recognised as one of the most important advances in the field of dementia care (Woods, 2001). Central to Kitwood's (1997, p.89) argument is the belief that 'positive person work' can do much to restore 'personhood' and enhance experiences of life, and the contribution that people can make. He recognised that personhood is socially constructed within relationships, with the challenge being to promote well-being through authentic partnerships (Dupuis *et al.*, 2011), requiring a collective effort to maintain the identity of the person living with dementia (Van Gennip *et al.*, 2014).

Support for Kitwood's thesis is provided by comprehensive reviews of the growing literature, such as that undertaken by Woods (2012), which conclude unequivocally that the quality of life of people living with dementia bears no relationship to the severity of their condition, but that one of the key factors is their relationships with others. However, it is on the nature and importance of such relationships that Kitwood's work is, perhaps, less well developed. This was recognised in a volume that sought both to bring Kitwood's collective writings together for a wider audience and to provide a critical commentary on his contribution to advancing the field (Baldwin and Capstick, 2007).

In critiquing Kitwood's concept of personhood, the editors of that volume argue that his vision is perhaps somewhat one-sided in that it sees personhood as something conferred on people *by others* in the context of relationships but does not explicitly acknowledge the part that the person living with dementia may play in conferring personhood *on others* (our emphasis). They sum this up as follows:

> Although the proposed theory of personhood is relational, Kitwood only captures a unidirectional realisation of that theory. Consequently, the theory and its realisation in person-centred care are individualistic and focussed on the person living with dementia to the exclusion of those caring for that person living with dementia. Thus the theory is uneven in the sense that people living with dementia have personhood bestowed on them but are not seen as bestowing personhood on others. They are thus made more dependent on and vulnerable to the vicissitudes of others. (Baldwin and Capstick, 2007)

Moreover, whilst Kitwood (1997, pp.7–19) stresses that people with dementia matter, he did not fully explore their potential to be active agents with multiple social roles, and his gaze does not stretch much beyond micro-social relationships (largely in a residential setting). He thereby does not fully explore the extent to which the experiences of people who have dementia are shaped by the socio-political context, nor the degree to which they can influence that context themselves (Baldwin and Capstick 2007).

More recent work has begun to redress the balance, according people living with dementia a more active role by highlighting the contribution that they can make. Central to this is the belief that people with dementia are able to reciprocate in multiple ways. For example, in describing their efforts to create 'authentic partnerships' with people who are living with dementia, Dupuis and colleagues (2011) stress the importance of 'synergistic relationships' in which interdependency and reciprocity are essential to ensuring that the contribution of everyone, especially the person who has dementia, is recognised and promoted. In considering the personal dignity of the person, Van Gennip and colleagues (2014) talk about the need to preserve identity and self at three levels:

- The 'inter-personal dimension' in which it is vital to create an environment in which people can still engage in meaningful activity.

- The 'relational-self' and the importance of facilitating interactions in which, although perhaps increasingly dependent on others, people living with dementia are still able to reciprocate.

- The 'social-self', comprising interactions with the outside world. This is seen as the most challenging arena, and the one in which a negative experience has the greatest potential to reduce dignity.

Maintaining a sense of 'social worth' and being able to engage with others is of great significance to people who are living with dementia, with Robertson (2014, p.538) stressing the need to both build on prior relationships and develop new ones: 'Finding meaning (when living with dementia) therefore depends on maintaining connections with valued roles and relationships from the past and establishing roles and relationships that bring a new sense of purpose to life.' This is not to say that people with dementia remain passive partners in the whole enterprise of establishing and maintaining positive relationships. It is within the literature around couplehood that we are able to discern the efforts made by people with dementia to maintain a sense of shared identity for spousal couples. For example, in Keady and Nolan's model of the dynamics of dementia, people with dementia were, in the most positive situations, identified as equal partners in 'working together' to 'make the best' of their situation (Keady and Nolan, 2003). Hellström, Nolan and Lundh (2007) were also able to point to the contribution made by people with dementia to 'sustaining couplehood', through continuing to talk about things on a shared basis as well as playing an active role in making the best of each day. More recently, Molyneaux and colleagues (2012) have also highlighted the role played by people with dementia in sustaining couplehood, particularly by maintaining shared activities. In their synthesis of qualitative research into relationships in dementia, La Fontaine and Oyebode (2014) stress the importance of long-term commitment and a 'shared history' as key to maintaining positive relationships, whilst also recognising that the nature of these relationships will change over time.

If we are therefore to both recognise the importance of relationships for a positive psychology of dementia and to realise the potential of such relationships, we need to expand our conceptual horizons.

Close relationships are a vital aspect of positive psychology. Peterson and Seligman (2004) describe strengths of humanity as those positive traits that manifest in caring relationships, describing these strengths as both interpersonal and social. Of these strengths, which also include kindness and social intelligence, perhaps the most fundamental is love, which occurs in reciprocal relationships that involve the sharing of comfort and acceptance. Communicating and receiving love deeply embodies acceptance, respect and care. Indeed, as Hendrick and Hendrick (2009, p.472) ask: 'What is more important than love for a happy life?' Altruism and compassion, as positive personal strengths or social processes, are additional concepts that are potentially relevant to further understanding positive close relationships in dementia.

Our vision of relationships must also be underpinned by the core values of interdependence and reciprocity (as opposed to dependence/independence and autonomy), in which the needs of all participants are fully acknowledged and accorded status (Nolan *et al.*, 2004). In addition, we must recognise that positive relationships exist at multiple levels, from very close interpersonal ties to more distant relationships with the wider community and society as a whole. Moreover, relationships are not just concerned with the people with whom we have contact but also the institutions, such as health and social care, with which we interact. In the remainder of this chapter we briefly explore how we might achieve this vision of interdependence and reciprocity.

INTERDEPENDENCE, RELATIONSHIPS AND DEMENTIA: CREATING AN ENRICHED ENVIRONMENT

At the end of their five-year programme 'A Better Life', exploring what quality of life means to people with high support needs, the Joseph Rowntree Foundation, as previously mentioned, identified seven key challenges (Blood, 2013). The central role accorded to relationships has already been alluded to, but also key is the need to treat all people as 'citizens' and to adopt an asset-based approach that recognises people's strengths and resources and creates opportunities for them to both give and receive support. Such arguments apply equally to people living with dementia, as is clear in recent initiatives such as the promotion of 'Dementia Friendly Communities' (Alzheimer's Society, 2013).

As we have argued, if such communities are to be created, there is a need to adopt a more inclusive definition of relationships that extends beyond the interpersonal. This is clearly recognised in initiatives such as 'Dementia without Walls' (Joseph Rowntree Foundation, 2014), predicated on the belief that we not only need to connect 'people with people' but also with the wider community. However, it is recognised that this will not be easy as it means 'fundamentally reshaping the *relationship* between individuals, the community and the state' (Joseph Rowntree Foundation, 2014, our emphasis).

If the above are to be achieved, there is for us an essential prior step, and that is to shift the rhetoric and the aspiration away from person-centred care to a more explicitly relational model (Nolan *et al.*, 2004). The debt that dementia care owes to Tom Kitwood has already been acknowledged, but with his work came the hegemony of a 'person-centred' model. This vision has now spread so far beyond dementia care that a confederation of 140 of the UK's leading charities has called for all health and social care to become person-centred by 2020 (National Voices, 2014). Person-centred care, consistent with Kitwood's original thesis, is essentially an individualistic approach and fails to recognise and address the necessary interdependencies that lie at the heart of all relationships. To our mind, its wholesale adoption will do little to improve, and indeed may exacerbate, existing tensions.

The need for an alternative model of care provision, particularly one that can meet the challenges posed by the rise in long-term conditions, was recognised some two decades ago by a major task force considering the future of healthcare in the USA (Tresolini and the Pew-Fetzer Task Force, 1994). They concluded that any effective system for the future must be based on a relationship-centred model that explicitly acknowledges that 'the interactions amongst people (are) the foundation of any therapeutic or healing activity' (Tresolini and the Pew-Fetzer Task Force, 1994, p.11). The concept of relationship-centred care (RCC) emerged as a consequence. However, whilst the task force provided a broad conceptual vision of what RCC might look like, they did not, as they acknowledge, propose a means by which such a model might be realised in practice.

To fill this gap, extensive work conducted over a 15-year period resulted in the initial development, refinement and application of a framework for RCC: 'The Senses Framework' (Nolan *et al.*, 2006). At the heart of the framework lies the goal of creating an 'enriched environment'. Such an environment is one in which *all* those involved experience six 'senses' (Nolan, 1997), as illustrated in Table 10.1.

Table 10.1: The six senses in the context of caring relationships

A SENSE OF SECURITY	
For older people	Attention to essential physiological and psychological needs, to feel safe and free from threat, harm, pain and discomfort. To receive competent and sensitive care.
For staff	To feel free from physical threat, rebuke or censure. To have secure conditions of employment. To have the emotional demands of work recognised and to work within a supportive but challenging culture.
For family carers	To feel confident in knowledge and ability to provide good care (To do caring well – Schumacher *et al.*, 1998) without detriment to personal well-being. To have adequate support networks and timely help when required. To be able to relinquish care when appropriate.
A SENSE OF CONTINUITY	
For older people	Recognition and value of personal biography; skilful use of knowledge of the past to help contextualise present and future. Seamless, consistent care delivered within an established relationship by known people.
For staff	Positive experience of work with older people from an early stage of career, exposure to good role models and environments of care. Expectations and standards of care communicated clearly and consistently.
For family carers	To maintain shared pleasures/pursuits with the care recipient. To be able to provide competent standards of care, whether delivered by self or others, to ensure that personal standards of care are maintained by others, to maintain involvement in care across care environments as desired/appropriate.
A SENSE OF BELONGING	
For older people	Opportunities to maintain and/or form meaningful and reciprocal relationships, to feel part of a community or group as desired.

For staff	To feel part of a team with a recognised and valued contribution, to belong to a peer group, a community of gerontological practitioners.
For family carers	To be able to maintain/improve valued relationships, to be able to confide in trusted individuals to feel that you're not 'in this alone'.
A SENSE OF PURPOSE	
For older people	Opportunities to engage in purposeful activity facilitating the constructive passage of time, to be able to identify and pursue goals and challenges, to exercise discretionary choice.
For staff	To have a sense of therapeutic direction, a clear set of goals to which to aspire.
For family carers	To maintain the dignity and integrity, well-being and 'personhood' of the care recipient, to pursue (re) constructive/reciprocal care (Nolan *et al.*, 1996).
A SENSE OF ACHIEVEMENT	
For older people	Opportunities to meet meaningful and valued goals, to feel satisfied with one's efforts, to make a recognised and valued contribution, to make progress towards therapeutic goals as appropriate.
For staff	To be able to provide good care, to feel satisfied with one's efforts, to contribute towards therapeutic goals as appropriate, to use skills and ability to the full.
For family carers	To feel that you have provided the best possible care, to know you've 'done your best', to meet challenges successfully, to develop new skills and abilities.
A SENSE OF SIGNIFICANCE	
For older people	To feel recognised and valued as a person of worth, that one's actions and existence are of importance, that you 'matter'.
For staff	To feel that gerontological practice is valued and important, that your work and efforts 'matter'.
For family carers	To feel that one's caring efforts are valued and appreciated, to experience an enhanced sense of self.

(From Nolan et al., 2006, pp.35–36, reproduced with permission)

Although originally developed for application in care home settings – the model now underpins major national initiatives in this sector such as 'My Home Life' (Age UK) – the framework has since been applied in a range of environments, including acute hospital care (Davies *et al.*, 1999; Patterson *et al.*, 2011) and the community, especially in services for people who are living with dementia and their family carers (Ryan *et al.*, 2004, 2008). It is this model that underpins our vision of how to realise the potential of positive relationships in dementia by creating an enriched environment throughout the dementia journey.

ENRICHING THE DEMENTIA EXPERIENCE: A TEMPORAL APPROACH

Whilst each individual experiences dementia in a unique way, over the last 15 years or so a number of models have emerged that see the experience as a 'journey' that unfolds over time and in which the needs of those involved vary depending on the stage of their journey. These so-called 'temporal' models have also changed in emphasis. Early attempts focused primarily on the experiences of family carers, with the voice of people who have dementia, to the extent that it was considered at all, being peripheral and based on proxy accounts provided by the carer (see Keady and Nolan, 2003). As a counter to this, later studies attempted to give a voice to people themselves, independent from that of the carer. More recently, dyadic models have emerged that attempt to capture the interactions between the person with dementia and their main carers, and that recognise both as active participants in shaping the experience of living with dementia (for a review, see La Fontaine and Oyebode, 2014). Building on this work, others are now promoting a family-centred approach that recognises the multiplicity of people involved in many situations (Roach et al., 2014).

Our vision of RCC, whilst being operationalised via the Senses Framework, is also underpinned by Rolland's vision of a 'therapeutic quadrangle' (Rolland, 1994). Rolland, an American psychologist, was primarily interested in the diversity of what used to be called 'chronic' illnesses and are now more commonly known as 'long-term conditions'. Rolland argued that chronic illnesses are infinitely more varied than acute ones, and the type of demands that they pose for all concerned will vary depending on:

- the nature of their onset

- the course that they run

- the degree of incapacity that they cause and when this manifests itself

- the eventual outcome and the likelihood of death.

So, for example, stroke usually has a rapid and unexpected onset, but after the initial period the course and incapacity are clearer and the likelihood of death diminishes (unless there is another stroke). In contrast, a condition like dementia has a very varied onset and course, which is usually more gradual but unpredictable, as is the timing of any incapacity and the likelihood of death.

For Rolland, an appropriate response to any condition will depend on the nature of the condition itself (as defined above) and the reactions of, and interactions between, the person living with the condition, his/her informal support and the 'system' (comprising both the individuals within it and its various processes and structures) providing more formal support. The sudden and unexpected nature of conditions such as a stroke initially makes multiple demands on the person with the stroke and their informal support, who are expected to 'learn' how to both live with the condition and 'manage' the system rapidly. Sadly, as multiple studies attest (for a review, see Nolan, 2001): rehabilitation is focused primarily on short-term physical recovery, with longer-term needs largely ignored; carers' needs are rarely considered a priority; and in the longer-term, dealing with the system often causes more problems than the presenting condition itself.

In contrast, a condition such as dementia typically manifests itself much more gradually, so by the time 'formal' help from the system is sought both the person and the carer may have lived with dementia for a considerable period of time and have expertise and insights of their own. This is often not acknowledged, and whilst things may have improved over time people's first contact with the system is often not a positive one and receiving a diagnosis is still largely a traumatic and stressful period operating within an impoverished environment (see Keady and Nolan, 2013).

Our approach to RCC seeks not to apportion blame but rather to understand why, despite decades of research and numerous policy initiatives, things seem slow to improve or are even getting worse, as the Francis report (2013) starkly highlights. It is clear that in many cases an 'enriched' environment is not created either for people with dementia or their family carers. However, one important question to consider is this: 'If staff do not experience an enriched work environment themselves, then is it possible for them to create such an environment for others?'

In a system where both significance and achievement are measured primarily in terms of meeting 'targets', and punitive measures are applied if such targets are not met, then the 'purpose' of care becomes distorted and lost. Priority is given to cure not care, and a short-term fix takes precedence over a longer-term solution. Staff do not feel secure enough to raise their concerns, being only too aware of what happens to 'whistle blowers'. Once established, an impoverished environment, in which the 'senses' are absent for one or more groups, becomes very difficult to shift, as the extensive literature on organisational change amply demonstrates. This is not to promote a counsel of despair but rather to recognise, as Held (2002, 2004) argues, that we have to openly acknowledge the 'negative side' of things if we are to have a balanced debate and to move forward. Taking Rolland's (1994) arguments, it is clear that all too often the system is focused primarily on meeting outcomes that have been largely defined for the benefit of the 'system', and are easy to measure rather than the subtler and diffuse needs of the person and their carer(s). If things are to improve, we need to focus on the benefits of positive relationships in dementia care and to highlight the advantages of creating an enriched environment, not only for people living with dementia but for all involved, whether in a family or a paid capacity.

Not surprisingly, although adequate resources and funding are important, an enriched environment turns more often on seemingly insignificant but subtle and vitally important forms of interaction, as well as the adoption of ways of working and systems of reward that see such forms of 'relational practice' as essential to good care (for an expanded version of these arguments, see Dewar and Nolan, 2013; Patterson *et al.*, 2011). Whilst space precludes a full description of these practices here, interested readers can access a wide range of sources exploring how to create the senses in a diverse array of settings including: care homes, acute care settings (Davies *et al.*, 1999; Patterson *et al.*, 2011), and the community (Ryan *et al.*, 2004, 2008), as well as the forms of 'caring conversations' that open up the type of dialogue needed to lay the foundations of an enriched environment (Dewar and Nolan, 2013). It is hoped that the case study below will provide a flavour of this.

SHINDIG – an 'enriched' support group for people living with dementia and family carers

Attending a support group has long been promoted as a means of living more positively with a long-term condition. Building on the notion of survivorship, it is argued that support groups enable people to share experiences and problem-solve within a safe reflective space. These are things that people living with dementia and their carers would clearly benefit from and, consequently, peer networks for these groups have been established across the UK. One such group, the Sheffield Dementia Involvement Group (SHINDIG), an alliance of people with dementia and family carers which is supported by a group of paid and volunteer supporters, was established in 2013. SHINDIG aims to promote the exchange of information and knowledge and has established itself as not only a place for the sharing of ideas and experiences, but also as a forum to help inform and shape local support services. As such, it provides the 'formal system' with an important source of expertise. However, and perhaps more importantly, it has become a place for potentially isolated people to build relationships.

People with dementia who are members of SHINDIG speak of the importance it now plays in their lives, especially as a place where they feel safe – not only to talk about their fears but also to laugh with one another about the world in which they live. Central to this are the warm and close relationships that exist within the group, with people living with dementia being central to creating such relationships. Here they don't feel like the 'odd one out'; rather they feel secure and that they belong, and the meetings create a sense of continuity, purpose and significance for them.

For the group's family caregivers, SHINDIG has also become an important part of their lives. Attending provides them with a rare comradery born out of having lived with similar challenges. Exchanging their experiences reinforces the significance of what they do; and sharing their expertise with service providers also helps to ensure that support for the person living with dementia is sensitive and appropriate, greatly enhancing carers' sense of purpose and achievement. That they can attend SHINDIG knowing that the person with dementia is also enjoying themselves creates a true 'win/win' scenario.

Such an 'enriched environment' takes considerable time, energy and skill to both create and sustain. Real expertise is required to help ensure that all attendees feel safe and secure to express their feelings and, on occasion, to engage in 'difficult' conversations. Facilitators and supporters are rightly proud of their work but recognise that the success of SHINDIG relies on a network of practitioners who share ideas, reflect regularly on what they do and seek to improve the way things work. Staff therefore not only create an 'enriched environment' but also enjoy one, with their efforts being fully recognised by the people with dementia and family caregivers who ensure that SHINDIG is a genuinely reciprocal and positive experience for all involved.

Whilst in no way providing a panacea, nor a quick, easy solution, we believe that adopting a relational approach to dementia care is one way of making a positive psychology of dementia, as reflected in an enriched environment and captured by the senses, much more achievable. However, to have any chance of success, we need to adopt the expanded view of relationships outlined above – one that extends our vision beyond the interpersonal to include relationships between the systems and structures of the organisations providing support and the wider society of which they are part. Only in this way will idea(l)s such as a 'dementia-friendly community' move beyond rhetoric.

For Gwen Mai Nolan (1931–2015), who enriched the lives of all she met.

REFERENCES

Alzheimer's Society (2013) 'Building dementia-friendly communities: A priority for everyone.' Available at www.alzheimers.org.uk/site/scripts/download_info.php?fileID=1916, accessed on 21 April 2016.

Aspinwall, L. and Tedeschi, R.G. (2010) 'The value of positive psychology for health psychology: Progress and pitfalls in examining the relationship of positive phenomena to health.' *Annals of Behavioral Medicine* 39(1), 4–15.

Baldwin, C. and Capstick, A. (2007) *Tom Kitwood on Dementia: A Reader and Critical Commentary*. Maidenhead: Open University Press.

Baltes, P. and Baltes, M. (1990) 'Psychological Perspectives on Successful Aging: The Model of Selective Optimization with Compensation.' In P. Baltes and M. Baltes (eds) *Successful Aging: Perspectives from the Behavioral Sciences*. Cambridge: University of Cambridge Press.

Blane, D., Wiggins, R.D., Montgomery, S.M., Hildon, Z. and Netuuel, G. (2012) *Resilience and Older Age: The Importance of Social Relationships and Implications for Policy*. International Centre for Life Course Studies, UCL, Paper 3.

Blood, I. (2013) *A Better Life: Valuing Our Later Years*. York: Joseph Rowntree Foundation.

Carstenson, L., Isaacowitz, D. and Charles, S. (1999) 'Taking time seriously: A theory of socioemotional selectivity theory.' *American Psychologist 54*(3),165–181.

Cumming, E. and Henry, W. (1961) *Growing Old: The Process of Disengagement*. New York, NY: Basic Books.

Davies, S., Nolan, M.R., Brown, J. and Wilson, F. (1999) *Good Practice in the Hospital Care of Older People*. London: Help the Aged.

Dewar, B. and Nolan, M.R. (2013) 'Caring about caring: Developing a model to implement compassionate relationship centred care in an older people care setting.' *International Journal of Nursing Studies 50*(9), 1247–1258.

Dupuis, S.L., Gillies, J., Carson, J., Whyte, C. *et al.* (2011) 'Moving beyond patient and client approaches: Mobilizing *"authentic partnerships"* in dementia care, support and services.' *Dementia 11*(4), 427–452.

Francis, R. (2013) *Report of the Mid Staffordshire NHS Foundation Trust Public Inquiry*. London: The Stationery Office.

Havighurst, R.J. (1963) 'Successful Aging.' In R. Williams, C. Tibbits and W. Donahue (eds) *Processes of Aging (Vol. 1)*. New York, NY: Atherton Press.

Hellström, I, Nolan, M. and Lundh, U. (2007) 'Sustaining "couplehood": Spouses' strategies for living positively with dementia.' *Dementia 6*(3), 383–409.

Held, B.S. (2002) 'The tyranny of positive attitudes in America: Observation and speculation.' *Journal of Clinical Psychology 58*, 651–669.

Held, B.S. (2004) 'The negative side of positive psychology.' *Journal of Humanistic Psychology 44*(1), 9–46.

Hendrick, C. and Hendrick, S.S. (2009) 'Love.' In S.J. Lopez and C.R. Snyder (eds) *The Oxford Handbook of Positive Psychology*. Oxford University Press, NY: New York.

Janssen, B.M., Van Regenmortel, T. and Abma, T.A. (2011) 'Identifying sources of strength: Resilience from the perspectives of older people receiving long-term community care.' *European Journal of Ageing 8*(3), 145–156.

Joseph Rowntree Foundation (2014) *Dementia Without Walls*. Available at http://dementiawithoutwalls.org.uk, accessed on 1 December 2015.

Katz, J., Holland, C, Peace, S. and Taylor, E. (2011) *A Better Life – What Older People With High Support Needs Value*. York: Joseph Rowntree Foundation.

Keady, J. and Nolan, M. (2003) 'The Dynamics of Dementia: Working Together, Working Separately, or Working Alone?' In M. Nolan, U. Lundh, G. Grant and J. Keady (eds) *Partnerships in Family Care: Understanding the Caregiving Career*. Maidenhead: Open University Press.

Keady, J. and Nolan, M. (2013) 'Person and Relationship Centred Care: Past, Present and Future.' In T. Dening and A.Thomas (eds) *Oxford Textbook on Old Age Psychiatry*. Oxford: Oxford University Press.

Kitwood, T. (1997) *Dementia Reconsidered: The Person Comes First*. Buckingham: Open University Press.

La Fontaine, J. and Oyebode, J. (2014) 'Family relationships and dementia: A synthesis of qualitative research including the person with dementia.' *Ageing and Society* 34(7), 1243–1272.

Lang, F.R. (2001) 'Regulation of social relationships in later adulthood.' *The Journals of Gerontology Series B: Psychological Sciences and Social Sciences* 56(6), 321–326.

Mercer, J. (1944) 'Ac-Cent-Tchu-ate the Positive.' MGM Records.

Minkler, M. (1996) 'Critical perspectives on ageing: New challenges for gerontology.' *Ageing and Society* 16(4), 467–487.

Molyneaux, V., Butchard, S., Simpson, J. and Murray, C. (2012) 'The co-construction of couplehood in dementia.' *Dementia* 11(4), 483–502.

National Voices (2014) Person centred care 2020: Calls and contributions from health and social care charities. Available at www.nationalvoices.org.uk/sites/default/files/public/publications/person-centred-care-2020.pdf, accessed on 22 April 2016.

Nolan, M.R. (1997) Health and social care: What the future holds for nursing. Plenary presentation at 3rd RCN Older Persons European Conference and Exhibition, The Old Swan, Harrogate (5 November 1997).

Nolan, M.R. (2001) 'Acute and Rehabilitative Care for Older People.' In M.R. Nolan, S. Davies and G. Grant (eds) *Working with Older People and Their Families: Key Issues for Policy and Practice*. Buckingham: Open University Press.

Nolan, M. R., Brown, J., Davies, S., Nolan, J. and Keady, J. (2006) *The Senses Framework: Improving Care for Older People through a Relationship-centred Approach*. Getting Research into Practice (GRiP) Report No 2, University of Sheffield.

Nolan, M.R., Davies, S., Brown, J., Keady, J. and Nolan, J. (2004) 'Beyond "person-centred" care: A new vision for gerontological nursing.' *International Journal of Older People Nursing* 13(3a), 45–53.

Nolan, M.R., Grant G. and Keady J. (1996) *Understanding Family Care*. Buckingham: Open University Press.

Nolan, M.R., Ryan, T., Enderby, P. and Reid, D. (2002) 'Towards a more inclusive vision of dementia care practice and research.' *Dementia* 1(2), 193–211.

Patterson, M., Nolan, M., Rick, J., Brown, J., Adams, R. and Musson, G. (2011) *From metrics to meaning: Culture change and quality of acute hospital care for older people*. Final report to NCCSDO. Available at www.nets.nihr.ac.uk/__data/assets/pdf_file/0003/64497/FR-08-1501-93.pdf, accessed on 22 April 2016.

Peterson, C. and Seligman, M.E.P. (2004) *Character Strengths and Virtues: A Handbook and Classification*. New York, NY: Oxford University Press.

Ranzijn, R. (2002a) 'Towards a positive psychology of ageing: Potentials and barriers.' *Australian Psychologist* 37(2) 79–85.

Ranzijn, R. (2002b) 'The potential of older adults to enhance community quality of life: Links between positive psychology and productive aging.' *Ageing International* 27(2), 30–55.

Roach, P., Keady, J., Bee, P. and Williams, S. (2014) '"We can't keep going on like this": Identifying family storylines in young onset dementia.' *Ageing and Society 34*, 1397–1426.

Roberts, Y. (2012) *One Hundred Not out: Resilience and Active Ageing*. Available at http://youngfoundation.org/wp-content/uploads/2012/10/100-Not-Out, accessed on 22 April 2016.

Robertson, J.M. (2014) 'Finding meaning in everyday life with dementia: A case study.' *Dementia 13*(4), 525–543.

Rolland, J.S. (1994) *Families, Illness and Disabilities: An Integrative Treatment Model*. New York, NY: Basic Books.

Rowe, J.W. and Kahn, R.L. (1987) 'Human aging: Usual and successful.' *Science 237*, 143–149.

Ryan, T., Nolan, M., Enderby, P. and Reid, D. (2004) '"Part of the family": Sources of job satisfaction amongst a group of community based dementia care workers.' *Health and Social Care in the Community 12*(2), 111–118.

Ryan, T., Nolan, M.R., Reid, D. and Enderby, P. (2008) 'Using the Senses Framework to achieve relationship-centred dementia care services: A case example.' *Dementia 7*(1), 71–93.

Scheidt, R.J., Humphreys, D.R. and Yorgason, J.B. (1999) 'Successful ageing: What's not to like?' *Journal of Applied Gerontology 18*(8), 277–282.

Schumacher, K.L., Stewart, B.J. and Archbold, P.G. (1998) 'Conceptualisation and measurement of doing family caregiving well.' *Image – the Journal of Nursing Scholarship 30*, 63–70.

Tanner, D. (2010) *Managing the Ageing Experience: Learning from Older People*. Bristol: The Policy Press.

Tornstam, L. (2005) *Gerotranscendence – A Developmental Theory of Positive Aging*. New York, NY: Springer.

Tresolini, C.P. and the Pew-Fetzer Task Force (1994) *Health Professions, Education and Relationship-centred Care*. San Francisco, CA: Pew Fetzer Health Professions Commission.

Van Gennip, L.E., Pasman, R.W., Oosterveld-Vlug, M.G., Willems, D.L. and Onwuteaka-Philipsen, B.D. (2014) 'How dementia affects personal dignity: A qualitative study of individuals with mild to moderate dementia.' *Journals of Gerontology, Series B: Psychological and Social Sciences*. DOI:10.1093/geronb/gbu137.

Walker, A. (1981) 'Towards a political economy of old age.' *Ageing and Society 1*(1), 73–94.

Woods, R.T. (2001) 'Discovering the person with Alzheimer's disease: Cognitive, emotional and behavioural aspects.' *Ageing and Mental Health 5*(1), S7–S16.

Woods, R.T. (2012) 'Well-being and dementia: How can it be achieved?' *Quality in Ageing and Older Adults*: 13(3), 205–211.

World Health Organization (WHO) (2002) *Active Ageing: A Policy Framework*. Available at www.who.int/ageing/publications/active_ageing/en, accessed on 22 April 2016.

Chapter 11

POSITIVE EXPERIENCES IN DEMENTIA CAREGIVING

Catherine Quinn

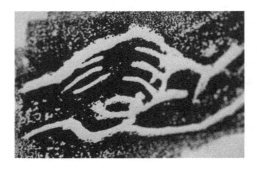

The term 'caregiver' has been used to describe a person who provides regular help and assistance to another person. This chapter focuses on informal dementia caregivers, who are usually family members or friends of the care recipient (i.e. the person living with dementia). In the UK, where approximately 61 per cent of people with dementia are living in the community and supported primarily by an informal caregiver, 44 per cent of the total cost of dementia to society is attributable to the cost of unpaid care. The total number of unpaid hours of care provided to people with dementia in the UK is worth £1.34 billion (Alzheimer's Society, 2014).

Many informal caregivers, particularly those in the earlier stages of caregiving, may not identify themselves as caregivers as they may feel they are simply helping out a family member or friend. Caregiving has been conceptualised as a career that begins as an individual is introduced to the caregiving role and that is marked by transitional events resulting in the gradual restructuring of the caregiver's self-concept around the caregiving role (Pearlin, 1992). This career continues through to the care recipient being placed into full-time residential care and beyond the death of the care recipient. Given the potentially longitudinal nature of dementia caregiving, it is important to understand the experience of caregiving so that effective support can be provided to caregivers where appropriate.

Caregiving has traditionally been perceived as an extremely stressful activity; indeed, studies have suggested that caregivers have worse health and well-being than non-caregivers (e.g. Pinquart and Sörenson, 2003). However, caregiving is a complex process and there are many factors that may influence how the caregiver responds to the challenges of caregiving. One way caregivers may adapt to these challenges is to identify positive aspects of providing care and the potential benefits of caregiving for either themselves or the care recipient or both. If caregivers can identify positives in their experience of providing care, then caregiving could be perceived as a source of gratification (Nolan, Grant and Keady, 1996).

This chapter will explore the positive aspects of providing care to a person living with dementia by first examining the role of positive emotions in challenging circumstances. It will provide examples of positive aspects of care identified in research with caregivers of older adults and people with other chronic health conditions. It will then explore the potential for dementia caregivers to identify and experience positive aspects of caregiving, using examples from research with informal caregivers providing care to people living with dementia.

POSITIVE EMOTIONS IN CHALLENGING CIRCUMSTANCES

People can experience high levels of stress whilst providing care for another person. Whilst this stress may suggest that caregiving is a negative experience, research indicates that both positive and negative psychological states can co-occur during challenging circumstances such as providing care (Folkman, 1997) and also that positive emotions have a significant role in how people respond and adjust to such experiences. Fredrickson and colleagues (2003) proposed that positive emotions provide an emotional break in a stressful situation and also replenish depleted resources. Whilst negative emotions might heighten our attention towards the need to deal with a threat, they can also narrow our thinking and behaviour. In contrast, positive emotions are involved in cognitive broadening, widening people's attention, thinking and behaviour (Fredrickson, 2004). This 'broaden and build' theory suggests that over time the broadening effect of positive emotions fosters the building of a range of adaptive and durable personal resources. Continuing opportunities to experience positive emotions will increase these resources, thus improving coping over the life-span and contributing to resilience – a person's ability to successfully adapt and cope with stressful situations.

As well as having a role in ongoing caregiving, positive emotions can also be important in motivating a person to provide help in the first place. Fredrickson (2004) proposed that experiencing positive emotions means a person is more likely to help someone, and, accordingly, this altruistic behaviour can result in gratitude in the person who was helped, leading to a reciprocation of help. Positive emotions may also have a role in maintaining caregivers' commitment to caregiving, as the ability to derive something positive out of caregiving could reinforce the desire to go on providing care. Caregivers may be motivated to provide care for altruistic or intrinsic reasons, where the desire is to help the care recipient. One key source of altruism is empathy, an emotional response to the perceived plight of another person. Feeling an empathetic emotion for someone in need can evoke an intrinsic, altruistic motivation to relieve that need by helping the person. At other times, helping behaviour may also be motivated by extrinsic factors, such as recognition from others (Batson *et al.*, 1991). It is possible that these different types of motivations occur at different times during caregiving as caregivers' motivations for sustaining caregiving change.

People might experience positive emotions in the face of adversity by finding meaning. The search for meaning is an integral aspect of people's lives and each individual's experience of meaning and its impact on coping and well-being may change over the course of the life-span (Zika and Chamberlain, 1992). Finding meaning may become more important in later life, as earlier sources of meaning – for instance, work or raising a family – can become less relevant (Coleman, 1995). Folkman (1997) distinguishes between two different types of meaning making. The first, global meaning, refers to a long-term belief system; the second, situational meaning, occurs in the context of a stressful event and describes the processes involved in assigning subjective meaning to that event (Park, 2010). Finding meaning after or in the midst of a stressful experience might help us to accept what has happened and even identify positive life changes (Park, 2010). Fredrickson (2004) has proposed that finding meaning should trigger positive emotions, but positive emotions should also broaden the likelihood of finding meaning.

The ability to transform adversity into something positive has also been referred to as 'benefit finding' (Baumeister and Vohs, 2002). Benefit finding may help people to adapt, and it has been linked to improved psychological and physical health (Tennen and Affleck, 2002). It has been suggested that benefit finding emerges over time in the process of adapting to adversity. In the short-term, benefit finding may be a technique for reducing distress and in the long-term it may reflect actual growth or change (Helgeson, Reynolds and Tomich, 2006). This may explain current inconsistent research findings on benefit finding, such as benefit finding being linked to poorer adjustment, as studies using cross-sectional designs have not been able to explore its development longitudinally (Tennen and Affleck, 2002). This has implications for research exploring positive benefits within the caregiving career.

POSITIVE ASPECTS OF CAREGIVING IN AGEING AND CHRONIC ILLNESS

Traditionally, caregiving research has tended to focus on the negative aspects of providing care, exploring outcomes such as burden or depression. Kramer (1997) identified that a lack of attention to positive aspects of caring in research has potentially skewed our perception of caregiving, limiting our understanding of how caregivers adapt. Kramer's early work on caregiving identified that in interviews caregivers often wanted to talk about various positive aspects of providing care, suggesting that this was an area that needed to be further explored. In a systematic review of gains in caregiving of older adults, Kramer (1997) identified 29 studies that used a variety of terms to describe gains in caregiving, such as satisfactions, uplifts, rewards, gratifications or benefits. Many of these terms lacked a theoretical background, thus it is difficult to determine whether these terms were synonymous. In light of these potential differences, in synthesising the literature for this chapter the term 'positive aspects of caregiving' (PAC) is used to describe positive features, processes and outcomes of caregiving.

The literature on PAC in ageing and chronic illness has key implications for exploring the role of positive aspects of dementia caregiving. Research with older adults has used both qualitative methodology, where the focus is on caregivers' descriptions of PAC, and quantitative methodology, where the focus is on factors that might be associated or predictive of caregivers' well-being. Noonan, Tennstedt and Rebelsky (1996) interviewed caregivers, who were either spouses, adult-children or other relatives, to explore meaning in caregiving. Caregiving was viewed as a source of gratification and satisfaction as it made them feel good and they felt their help was appreciated by the care recipient. Cohen, Colantonio and Vernich (2002) reported that, when asked, 73 per cent of spousal and family caregivers could identify PAC in their experiences. Commonly identified positive elements were that caregiving provided companionship, it was seen as fulfilling or rewarding, and that people enjoyed providing care. Findings from quantitative research further illustrate how PAC are associated with higher well-being, with lower burden, depression and poor health (Cohen et al., 2002). A lack of PAC can also have a detrimental impact on well-being as this is associated with negative emotional states such as burden, depression and anger (Lopez, Lopez-Arrieta and Crespo, 2005).

Several factors have been linked to PAC. Studies have considered the quality of the relationship between the caregiver and care recipient, with higher satisfaction in caregivers of older adults related to a better current and previous affective relationship (Iecovich, 2011; Lopez et al., 2005). The living situation of the care recipient may also be important. Pallant and Reid (2014) measured positive attitudes to caregiving in informal caregivers of older adults who either lived in the community or in a residential aged care facility (RACF). There was a significant difference in positive attitude between those caregivers whose care-recipients were in the community and those in a RACF, with more positive attitudes present in the RACF group.

Some studies have reported individual differences in PAC in caregivers of older adults. Lopez, Lopez-Arrieta and Crespo (2005) found that men reported more PAC than women, and both adult-children and spouses identified more PAC than other types of relationships (e.g. sons-in-law). However, other studies have not found any gender differences (e.g. Pallant and Reid, 2014). Broese van Groenou, de Boer and Iedema (2013) explored kin-relationship differences in PAC. For spouses, higher levels of PAC were associated with being motivated to provide care to prevent residential care admission and a stronger preference for informal care. In contrast, for adult-children being female, being motivated to provide care due to a strong bond with the care recipient as well as stronger preferences for informal care were associated with higher PAC. In addition, in this group higher levels of PAC were associated with providing more hours of care and the care recipient having more physical limitations, but fewer challenging behaviours.

Although the literature on caregiving in older adults highlights the potential role of PAC in dementia caregiving, there are differences between providing care to an older adult and someone living with dementia. Dementia is a chronic progressive condition and it is therefore useful to explore the literature on PAC in other chronic conditions. Folkman's (1997) early work with caregivers of people living with AIDS found that they experienced high levels of positive psychological states during the course of caregiving and bereavement. These positive psychological states were considered to be a form of coping; the caregivers coped through positive re-appraisal and infusing ordinary events, such as going to the cinema, with meaning. Carlisle (2000) also reported that caregivers of people living with HIV and AIDS could positively re-appraise the situation by identifying personal growth. Caregivers found meaning in the care recipient's condition by accepting the presence of the virus and by having a positive attitude.

Haley and colleagues (2009) found that family caregivers of people who had experienced a stroke reported that caregiving made them feel needed and strengthened their relationship with others. It also gave them a purpose and helped them to appreciate life more. Similarly, in a systematic review of positive caregiving experiences following stroke, Mackenzie and Greenwood (2012) identified how providing care can give meaning and purpose to caregivers' lives, improve their relationship with the care recipient and make them feel a better person. The findings from the included longitudinal studies also suggested that caregivers identified more PAC over time, suggesting that the ability to identify PAC may gradually occur. This may echo research findings on benefit finding in adversity, as described above.

A degenerative condition similar to dementia is Parkinson's disease. Habermann and Davis (2005) compared caregivers of people living with Alzheimer's disease and caregivers of people living with Parkinson's disease. In response to open-ended questions, caregivers of people living with Alzheimer's disease described sources of satisfaction, such as feeling appreciated, feeling positive that they were able to help and being together with the care recipient. Caregivers of people living with Parkinson's disease described positive aspects, such as knowing the care recipient was receiving good care and feeling that they were helping the family. They were able to identify more satisfactions than caregivers of people living with Alzheimer's disease, suggesting differences due to the condition of the care recipient. In both groups there were caregivers who could not identify any PAC, which suggests that there will be differences in the characteristics of people who identify PAC and those who do not.

CAN PROVIDING CARE TO A PERSON LIVING WITH DEMENTIA BE A POSITIVE EXPERIENCE?

Dementia is a progressive degenerative condition and it is often assumed that providing care to a person with dementia is inevitably very stressful and only has a negative impact on caregivers' well-being. However, findings from qualitative research studies indicate that caregivers of people living with dementia also experience PAC. Reflecting the concepts of meaning-focused coping and benefit finding, some dementia caregivers reframe how they view the situation by adopting a positive attitude and focusing on blessings rather than losses (Shim et al., 2013). Others perceive caregiving as a form of personal growth, as they discover more about themselves through caregiving, becoming a better person and learning new skills (Netto, Jenny and Philip, 2009; Shim et al., 2013; Quinn, Clare and Woods, 2015). Caregivers have described developing a sense of competence in their role by finding ways of coping with difficult situations and deriving satisfaction from keeping the person living with dementia within the community (Cohen et al., 1994; Peacock et al., 2010). Others have found gains due to the strengthening of their relationship with the person living with dementia and being able to reciprocate past love and help (Netto et al., 2009; Shim et al., 2013; Quinn et al., 2015).

However, not all caregivers are able to identity experiencing PAC (e.g. Cohen et al., 1994) and, as yet, it is unclear to what extent PAC might affect outcomes for the care recipient. Research to date has been constrained by study designs as many are cross-sectional and it has been suggested that growth or benefit finding in caregiving may emerge later on in the process of adapting to stress (Helgeson *et al.*, 2006). It is also currently unclear exactly what role PAC has in the caregiving experience and there are some key questions to consider when thinking about the role of PAC in dementia caregiving, including:

- Are PAC linked to the negative outcomes of caregiving?

- What role do PAC play in the caregiving experience? What is the impact of experiencing PAC and what factors influence them?

- Should interventions be targeted at improving PAC?

- Do PAC influence outcomes for the person living with dementia?

The rest of this chapter will address some of these issues, highlighting gaps in current research. In order to explore research into PAC in dementia caregiving, it is important to first understand the theoretical models that have guided dementia caregiving research. These models highlight that there are multiple factors that can influence the caregiving experience and there are differences in how PAC has been incorporated into these models.

THEORETICAL MODELS OF DEMENTIA CAREGIVING

One of the dominant models influencing dementia caregiving research has been the Stress Process Model (SPM; Pearlin *et al.*, 1990), which acknowledges that caregiving is a complex process involving great variation in how a person adapts to and copes with the caregiving role. The central concept underlying the SPM is that caregiving is stressful. The SPM contains four main components: the background and context of stress, stressors, resources/mediators and outcomes. There is a dynamic relationship between stressors and resources, such as coping or social support, whereby effective resources may decrease the impact of stressors, whilst ineffective resources may increase stressors. The SPM has been criticised for primarily focusing on the negative consequences of caregiving. There is some recognition of gain but it is oddly encompassed under stressors, with the suggestion that gain involves enhancement of the self. The 'management of meaning' is also one of the techniques caregivers can use to cope with the stressors.

Whilst the SPM offers a useful framework to aid understanding of the role of multiple factors on the outcomes of caregiving, in order to develop our understanding of PAC in dementia caregiving, theoretical models of caregiving that explicitly incorporate the role of PAC need to be further developed. Two-factor models of caregiving acknowledge that caregiving could have both positive and negative outcomes. Lawton and colleagues (1991) conceived a two-factor model of caregiving appraisal, which proposed that caregiver burdens and satisfactions can have differential impacts on well-being, with caregiving satisfaction resulting in positive affect and caregiving burden resulting in negative affect. Similarly, Kramer (1997) proposed a conceptual model of caregiving in which appraisals of role gain result in positive outcomes and appraisals of role strain result in negative outcomes. Whilst both these models contain positive and negative aspects of caregiving, neither allows for negative aspects of care to have an impact on positive outcomes. It has been argued that positive and negative aspects of caregiving are different dimensions of the caregiving experience and that caregiving is neither a wholly negative nor positive experience (Broese van Groenou *et al.*, 2013; Iecovich, 2011).

ARE PAC LINKED TO NEGATIVE OUTCOMES OF CAREGIVING?

Whilst it is possible that positive and negative aspects of dementia caregiving are separate dimensions, some studies have found a relationship between them. For instance, Rapp and Chao (2000) developed a measure of caregiving appraisals to examine the relationship between caregiving strain and gain. They found that higher caregiving gain was significantly correlated with lower strain. Some studies have explored the relationship between PAC and caregiving burden (caregivers' subjective appraisal of the demands of caregiving). Burden is considered a potentially modifiable factor of caregiving, and many interventions have been designed to reduce the burden of caregiving. Some studies have found that PAC is related to burden, with higher PAC linked to lower burden (Cohen *et al.*, 1994; Gold *et al.*, 1995; Gonclaves-Pereira *et al.*, 2010; Lawton *et al.*, 1991; Monin, Schulz and Feeney, 2015; Quinn, Clare, McGuinness and Woods, 2012). However, there have been different conceptualisations of burden, resulting in mixed findings and suggesting complicated relationships between burden and PAC. Boerner, Schulz and Horowitz (2004) found that burden associated with memory and behaviour problems was negatively associated with caregiving benefit, but caregiving benefit was not related to burden associated with activities of daily living (ADL).

Depression is often seen as a negative outcome of caregiving, and some studies have found that PAC are linked to lower depression (Lawton *et al.*, 1991; Monin *et al.*, 2015; Semiatin and O'Connor, 2012). However, depression may not necessarily be an outcome of caregiving as depression can precede the commencement of caregiving. Links between PAC and negative aspects of care need to be explored further, particularly as to whether PAC mediates the negative impact of providing care or whether negative experiences result in positive meaning making over time (Noonan *et al.*, 1996).

WHAT ROLE DO PAC PLAY IN THE CAREGIVING EXPERIENCE?

The fact that some dementia caregivers, but not all, can identify PAC raises questions about the role PAC have in the caregiving experience. PAC have been measured and conceptualised in different ways, often lacking a theoretical background. They can be seen as fixed personal dispositions linked to factors such as the caregivers' gender or age (e.g. Kramer, 1993b). However, the available evidence strongly suggests that there are factors that can influence caregivers' abilities to identify PAC. In research, PAC have been conceptualised in different ways; as a mediator, in the form of a coping strategies, or as an outcome of caregiving.

Some studies have conceptualised PAC in relation to meaning making as a coping strategy. A systematic review on meaning in dementia caregiving found that finding meaning has a positive impact on caregiver well-being (Quinn, Clare and Woods, 2010). Gotlieb and Gignac (1996, p.152) found that meaning making was significantly more likely to be employed as a coping mechanism to deal with the symptoms of dementia than when dealing with the effects of the caregiver having to give up 'something valued or something they looked forward to' because of caregiving. Finding meaning was positively associated with caregivers' sense of coherence and a flexible and adaptive dispositional orientation, which has been linked to successful coping (Gallagher et al., 1994). Saad and colleagues (1995, p.495) found that caregivers who coped by reducing their expectations of the care recipient and constructing a 'larger sense of the illness' also had lower levels of depression.

Some studies have treated PAC in dementia as an outcome and have explored the predictors of it. Many factors have been identified as influencing PAC, although few have been studied consistently and existing studies have looked at a diverse range of variables so at this point it is difficult to gain an understanding of exactly which ones predict PAC. Kramer (1993b) reported that 31 per cent of variance in caregiving satisfaction in wife caregivers was explained by caregiving stressors, quality of the relationship and marital history and resources and appraisals. Only quality of the prior relationship and ADL significantly predicated caregiving satisfaction, thus a better quality of prior relationship and greater limitations in ADL were linked to greater caregiving satisfaction. Harwood and colleagues (2000) reported that 42 per cent of the variance in caregiving satisfaction was predicted by behavioural disturbances, age, gender, health and social support.

Some research has suggested that caregivers' motivations to provide care influence the ability to experience and identify PAC (Broese van Groenou et al., 2013). It is feasible that the reasons (negative or positive) why a caregiver commenced caregiving should be related to PAC. Quinn and colleagues (2015) reported that some caregivers found it difficult to find meaning (one potential component of PAC) in their role because of feeling trapped. Indeed, higher meaning has been found to be a significant predictor of greater feelings of role captivity, where the caregiver feels trapped in the caregiving role (Quinn, Clare, McGuinness and Woods, 2012). Quinn, Clare and Woods (2012) report that meaning is significantly predicted by high religiosity, high competence, high intrinsic motivations (internal desires to provide care) and low role captivity. Interestingly, higher meaning has also been linked to higher extrinsic motivations, which relate to extrinsic pressures to provide care, such as the expectations of others (Quinn, Clare and Woods, 2012). This implies that it is caregivers' awareness of their reasons for providing care that helps them find meaning in their role.

Research findings and conceptual accounts of caregiving both indicate that there may be a link between PAC and the quality of the caregivers' current and previous relationship with the person living with dementia (e.g. Kramer, 1993b). Findings from qualitative research have indicated that caregivers do derive satisfactions from their relationship with the person living with dementia (e.g. Quinn *et al.*, 2015), suggesting that, for some, reciprocity and meaningful relationships are preserved. Correspondingly, both a better pre-caregiving and current relationship quality have been linked to higher PAC (Quinn, Clare and Woods, 2012; Quinn, Clare, McGuinness and Woods, 2012). Some studies have found that relationship quality predicts variance in PAC (Kramer, 1993b), whilst other studies have not supported this trend (Quinn, Clare and Woods, 2012), suggesting the influence of other mediators. It may be that perceptions of change in the relationship are linked to PAC. Spouse caregivers who perceived a change in marital closeness had reductions in PAC, whereas perceived continuity in their relationship, even in couples who were not close, was associated with greater PAC (Motenko, 1989). Caregiving has also been linked to the caregivers' relationship with others and their support network. Higher PAC has been linked to greater social involvement, a wider social support network and higher satisfaction with this network (Gold *et al.*, 1995; Harwood *et al.*, 2000; Kramer, 1993a, 1993b).

Given these varied findings, there is an acknowledged need to build integrated conceptual accounts of PAC that go beyond stress-appraisal models and simplistic two-factor models of caregiving. On the basis of a systematic review of PAC, Carbonneau, Caron and Desrosiers (2010) developed a conceptual model that relates the likelihood of experiencing PAC to caregivers' feelings of self-efficacy as well as the quality of relationship with the person living with dementia. In this model, three key domains of PAC are delineated: the quality of the daily relationship between the caregiver and the care recipient, the meaning derived from the role of caregiving and also the caregiver's sense of accomplishment. These factors interact and influence outcomes of caregiving in terms of well-being and continuity of the role. They are seen as emerging through a combination of caregiver self-efficacy and the occurrence of daily 'enrichment' events, such as sharing a pleasant activity with the care recipient. Although this is only a conceptual framework, it does provide an indication of how components of PAC might interact and differ between individuals, whilst also suggesting *how* caregivers might find ways to go beyond coping and adjusting to dementia caregiving towards finding meaning, accomplishment and growth.

SHOULD INTERVENTIONS BE TARGETED AT IMPROVING PAC?

Few studies have explored PAC longitudinally and there certainly needs to be more research on how they might change throughout the caregiving career. It is important to acknowledge that identifying PAC is an individual process – not all caregivers will be able to identify PAC nor should they be expected to. Whilst interventions may not be able to directly enable caregivers to experience PAC, caregivers might be helped to appraise their situations more positively, which could eventually result in them experiencing caregiving more positively. As an example of this possibility, Cheng and colleagues (2014) piloted a new intervention that targeted benefit finding through positive appraisal coping. The intervention reduced dementia caregivers' levels of depression, although some caregivers found it difficult to grasp the concept of benefit finding.

Some research findings indicate that changes in the caregiving situation influence PAC. Savundranayagam (2014) found that increases in the amount of help received from others as well as satisfaction with this help were both associated with an increase in PAC in the form of positive attitudes towards the dementia caregiving role. Decreases in daily care burden have also been associated with increases in PAC (Hilgeman *et al.*, 2007). These findings suggest that interventions that alter the caregiving situation and reduce burden could potentially influence PAC. Other modifiable factors could also be targeted. As noted, for example, self-efficacy may be related to PAC (Carbonneau *et al.*, 2010; Semiatin and O'Connor, 2012). Related to self-efficacy, caregiving competence – how caregivers appraise their ability to perform their role – has also been linked to higher PAC (Quinn, Clare and Woods, 2012; Quinn, Clare, McGuinness and Woods, 2012). It is possible that interventions that increase feelings of caregiving competence will help to enable caregivers to find PAC. Interventions would also need to take into account other factors linked to PAC – for instance, interventions promoting PAC may be more successful if the caregiver has, and has had, a good relationship with the person living with dementia.

DO PAC INFLUENCE OUTCOMES FOR THE PERSON LIVING WITH DEMENTIA?

There has been very little research on the direct impact of caregivers identifying PAC on outcomes for the person living with dementia. Indirect effects may be inferred from the fact that if PAC reduces caregiver burden and increases their well-being then this may result in benefits for the person living with dementia. PAC could impact on the quality of care provided (Kramer, 1997) and this is certainly an area that requires further research. Some studies have explored the role of PAC in decisions about arranging residential care for the person living with dementia, with mixed findings. PAC has been linked to the caregiver making a decision, or expressing a desire, to place the care recipient into full-time residential care but 18 months later was not linked to actual placement (Cohen *et al.*, 1994). Pruncho, Michaels and Potashnik (1990) found that spousal caregivers who placed the care recipient into full-time care reported fewer uplifts than those who continued to provide care in the community.

Lived experiences of positive aspects of dementia caregiving

As part of a wider study exploring how meaning, motivation, and relationship dynamics influence caregivers' subjective experience of caregiving, family caregivers were interviewed about the meaning they found in dementia caregiving (for full details of the study see Quinn et al., 2015). Excerpts from interviews with two of the participants are presented here to illustrate the subjective experience of meaning making and PAC amongst informal caregivers.

Brenan was caring for his wife, who was in the later stages of dementia. Although he found caregiving challenging at times, he was able to derive a great deal of meaning from his role, feeling that caregiving had made him a better person:

> I've got satisfaction, I feel that I'm a better person, a more complete person so this helps one to balance it out. I mean I suppose initially I was extremely sad about what

had taken place but as the years have gone by I trust I've become a more sympathetic person to the situation.

Brenan also derived satisfaction from feeling he was fulfilling his marital duty – he felt it was his responsibility to provide care for his wife:

> Well it helps me to cope yes very much because...I get a satisfaction out of doing my duty.

> I think the satisfaction and enjoyment is based...as far as I am concerned more on duty and on [doing] what I promised when we got married.

In contrast to Brenan, Carol was providing care for her father, who had more advanced dementia. Similarly to Brenan, however, the meaning she derived from her role was linked to motivations to provide care, represented in a feeling that she was reciprocating past help as it was now 'payback time':

> He's always been a really good dad. I mean I think if he hadn't I wouldn't really [have] felt quite so obliged to do it, you know, but he's always been there for me and he's always supported me.

Carol felt positive because she was doing 'the right thing' for her father and she did not want to feel guilty for not providing care for him. Carol gained satisfaction from being able to care for her father at home and not having to place him into full-time care:

> [I'm] sort of taking a pride in just making sure he's properly looked after, you know; he's got clean sheets and he's not sort of left struggling to do his shoe laces up, you know; all those things give you a sense of satisfaction as well.

Although both Carol and Brenan could identify meaning in their role, this was not enough to completely mitigate the stresses of providing care. Carol was acutely aware that the situation might alter, and if her father deteriorated and became less aware, the caregiving situation might change.

SUMMARY

There is preliminary evidence that PAC can be identified by caregivers of people living with dementia and that experiencing PAC is linked with well-being. The majority of research on PAC in caregiving has used cross-sectional designs, and a wide variety of variables have been linked to PAC. However, there is a need for more longitudinal research to enrich our knowledge about PAC and to identify whether caregivers are more likely to identify PAC over time. There are some studies in progress that will be able to explore PAC longitudinally – for instance, the IDEAL study (Clare *et al.*, 2014) is examining factors linked to living well with dementia. In this study participants are followed up for three years and there is scope to explore the longitudinal impact of PAC on outcomes for both the caregiver and person living with dementia.

There is also a need for further research to address various gaps in the current literature. Critically, there has been very little research on the direct impact of PAC on outcomes (e.g. quality of life) for the person living with dementia. Other important avenues for further research include the need to develop more consistent conceptualisations and measures of PAC since many studies use different terminologies to refer to PAC and it is difficult to determine whether the measures used are conceptually different. This is also related to the fact that many studies in this area lack a theoretical background. Those studies that utilise caregiving models generally tend to focus on the negative consequences of caregiving. In addition, in models such as the SPM (Pearlin *et al.*, 1990), positive emotions are only seen to occur in response to stressful situations, yet it is feasible that positive emotions could be directly related to caregiving; a caregiver may not need to perceive the situation as stressful to experience positive emotions. Positive psychology models based on positive emotions, such as the 'broaden and build' theory (Frederickson, 2004), and conceptual accounts of PAC, draw links between key factors such as meaning making, positive emotion and resilience, and these could prove useful in explaining why some caregivers not only cope but also thrive in their role.

The impact of PAC on the dementia caregiving experience has important implications for the development and delivery of support services. In order for healthcare professionals and services to provide more effective support for caregivers, there needs to be a better understanding of PAC. Identifying the ways in which caregivers might feel enriched by caregiving will help healthcare professionals to appropriately validate caregivers' feelings and experiences (Kramer, 1997). Research on PAC can provide pointers on how to enhance it or identify caregivers who are in more need of intervention. Caregivers who cannot find PAC may be at greater risk of caregiving having a detrimental impact on their well-being. In addition, PAC may also be an important determinant of the quality of care provided (Kramer, 1997). Thus, those caregivers who cannot identify PAC may require additional support. However, it must also be recognised that not all caregivers will be able to identify PAC.

Whilst there needs to be further research into the role of PAC, existing research contests the notion that providing care for a person living with dementia is a wholly negative experience. There is both qualitative and quantitative evidence that caregivers can identify positive aspects in providing care. There will be individual differences in what these positive aspects are – for instance, some may describe personal growth, others may derive something positive out of maintaining their relationship with the person living with dementia. Research into PAC is extending our understanding of how caregivers adapt to caregiving and is challenging traditional discourses that dementia caregiving is a purely stressful and unrewarding experience.

For the preparation of this chapter I would like to gratefully acknowledge the support of the Economic and Social Research Council (UK) and the National Institute for Health Research (UK) through grant ES/L001853/1 'Improving the experience of dementia and enhancing active life: Living well with dementia' (Investigators: L. Clare, I.R. Jones, C. Victor, J.V. Hindle, R.W. Jones, M. Knapp, M. Kopelman, A. Martyr, F. Matthews, R.G. Morris, S.M. Nelis, J. Pickett, C. Quinn, J. Rusted, N. Savitch and J. Thom).

REFERENCES

Alzheimer's Society (2014) *Dementia UK: Update*. London: Alzheimer's Society.

Batson, C.D., Batson, J.G., Slingsby, J.K., Harrell, K.L., Peekna, H.M. and Todd, R.M. (1991) 'Empathic joy and the empathy-altruism hypothesis.' *Journal of Personality and Social Psychology 61*(3), 413–426.

Baumeister, R.F. and Vohs, K.D. (2002) 'The Pursuit of Meaningfulness in Life.' In C.R. Snyder and S.J. Lopez (eds) *Handbook of Positive Psychology*. New York, NY: Oxford University Press.

Boerner, K., Schulz, R. and Horowitz, A. (2004) 'Positive aspects of caregiving and adaptation to bereavement.' *Psychology and Aging 19*(4), 668–675.

Broese van Groenou, M.I., de Boer, A. and Iedema, J. (2013) 'Positive and negative evaluation of caregiving among three different types of informal care relationships.' *European Journal of Ageing 10*(4), 301–311.

Carbonneau, H., Caron, C. and Desrosiers, J. (2010) 'Development of a conceptual framework of positive aspects of caregiving in dementia.' *Dementia 9*(3), 327–353.

Carlisle, C. (2000) 'The search for meaning in HIV and AIDS: The carers' experience.' *Qualitative Health Research 10*(6), 750–765.

Cheng, S.T., Lau, R.W., Mak, E.P., Ng, N.S. and Lam, L.C. (2014) 'Benefit-finding intervention for Alzheimer caregivers: Conceptual framework, implementation issues, and preliminary efficacy.' *The Gerontologist 54*(6), 1049–1058.

Clare, L., Nelis, S.M., Quinn, C., Martyr, A. *et al.* (2014) 'Improving the experience of dementia and enhancing active life – living well with dementia: Study protocol for the IDEAL study.' *Health and Quality of Life Outcomes 12*, 164.

Cohen, C.A., Colantonio, A. and Vernich, L. (2002) 'Positive aspects of caregiving: Rounding off the caregiving experience.' *International Journal of Geriatric Psychiatry 17*(2), 184–188.

Cohen, C.A., Gold, D.P., Shlman, K.I. and Zucchero, C.A. (1994) 'Positive aspects in caregiving: An overlooked variable in research.' *Canadian Journal on Aging 13*(3), 378–391.

Coleman, P.G. (1995) 'Facing the Challenges of Aging: Development, Coping and Meaning in Life.' In J.F. Nussbaum and J. Coupland (eds) *Handbook of Communication and Aging Research*. Hove: Lawrence Erlbaum Associates.

Folkman, S. (1997) 'Positive psychological states and coping with severe stress.' *Social Science and Medicine 45*(8), 1207–1221.

Fredrickson, B.L. (2004) 'The broaden-and-build theory of positive emotions.' *Philosophical Transactions of the Royal Society of London. Series B: Biological Sciences 359*(1449), 1367–1377.

Fredrickson, B.L., Tugade, M.M., Waugh, C.E. and Larkin, G.R. (2003) 'What good are positive emotions in crises? A prospective study of resilience and emotions following the terrorist attacks on the United States on September 11th, 2001.' *Journal of Personality and Social Psychology 84*(2), 365–376.

Gallagher, T.J., Wagenfeld, M.O., Baro, F. and Haepers, K. (1994) 'Sense of coherence, coping and caregiver role overload.' *Social Science and Medicine 39*(12), 1615–1622.

Gold, D.P., Cohen, C., Shulman, K., Zucchero, C., Andres, D. and Etezadi, J. (1995) 'Caregiving and dementia: Predicting negative and positive outcomes for caregivers.' *International Journal of Aging and Human Development 41*(3), 183–201.

Goncalves-Pereira, M., Carmo, I., da Silva, J.A., Papoila, A.L., Mateos, R. and Zarit, S.H. (2010) 'Caregiving experiences and knowledge about dementia in Portuguese clinical outpatient settings.' *International Psychogeriatrics 22*(2), 270–280.

Gottlieb, B.H. and Gignac, M.A.M. (1996) 'Content and domain specificity of coping among family caregivers of persons with dementia.' *Journal of Aging Studies 10*(2), 137–155.

Habermann, B. and Davis, L.L. (2005) 'Caring for family with Alzheimer's disease and Parkinson's disease: Needs, challenges, and satisfactions.' *Journal of Gerontological Nursing 31*(6), 49–54.

Haley, W.E., Allen, J.Y., Grant, J.S., Clay, O.J., Perkins, M. and Roth, D.L. (2009) 'Problems and benefits reported by stroke family caregivers: Results from a prospective epidemiological study.' *Stroke 40*(6), 2129–2133.

Harwood, D.G., Barker, W.W., Ownby, R.L., Bravo, M., Aguero, H. and Duara, R. (2000) 'Predictors of positive and negative appraisal among Cuban American caregivers of Alzheimer's disease patients.' *International Journal of Geriatric Psychiatry 15*(6), 481–487.

Helgeson, V.S., Reynolds, K.A. and Tomich, P.L. (2006) 'A meta-analytic review of benefit finding and growth.' *Journal of Consulting and Clinical Psychology 74*(5), 797–816.

Hilgeman, M.M., Allen, R.S., DeCoster, J. and Burgio, L.D. (2007) 'Positive aspects of caregiving as a moderator of treatment outcome over 12 months.' *Psychology and Aging 22*(2), 361–371.

Iecovich, E. (2011) 'Quality of relationships between care recipients and their primary caregivers and its effect on caregivers' burden and satisfaction in Israel.' *Journal of Gerontological Social Work 54*(6), 570–591.

Kramer, B.J. (1993a) 'Expanding the conceptualization of caregiver coping: The importance of relationship-focused coping strategies.' *Family Relations 42*(4), 383–391.

Kramer, B.J. (1993b) 'Marital history and the prior relationship as predictors of positive and negative outcomes among wife caregivers.' *Family Relations 42*(4), 367–375.

Kramer, B.J. (1997) 'Gain in the caregiving experience: Where are we? What next?' *The Gerontologist 37*(2), 218–232.

Lawton, M.P., Moss, M., Kleban, M.H., Glicksman, A. and Rovine, M. (1991) 'A two-factor model of caregiving appraisal and psychological well-being.' *Journal of Gerontology 46*(4), 181–189.

Lopez, J., Lopez-Arrieta, J. and Crespo, M. (2005) 'Factors associated with the positive impact of caring for elderly and dependent relatives.' *Archives of Gerontology and Geriatrics 41*(1), 81–94.

Mackenzie, A. and Greenwood, N. (2012) 'Positive experiences of caregiving in stroke: A systematic review.' *Disability and Rehabilitation 34*(17), 1413–1422.

Monin, J.K., Schulz, R. and Feeney, B.C. (2015) 'Compassionate love in individuals with Alzheimer's disease and their spousal caregivers: Associations with caregivers' psychological health.' *The Gerontologist 55*(6), 981–989.

Motenko, A.K. (1989) 'The frustrations, gratifications, and well-being of dementia caregivers.' *The Gerontologist 29*(2), 166–172.

Netto, N.R., Jenny, G.Y.N. and Philip, Y.L.K. (2009) 'Growing and gaining through caring for a loved one with dementia.' *Dementia 8*(2), 245–261.

Nolan, M., Grant, G. and Keady, J. (1996) *Understanding Family Care*. Buckingham: Open University Press.

Noonan, A.E., Tennstedt, S.L. and Rebelsky, F.G. (1996) 'Making the best of it: Themes of meaning among informal caregivers to the elderly.' *Journal of Aging Studies* 10(4), 313–327.

Pallant, J.F. and Reid, C. (2014) 'Measuring the positive and negative aspects of the caring role in community versus aged care setting.' *Australasian Journal on Ageing* 33(4), 244–249.

Park, C.L. (2010) 'Making sense of the meaning literature: An integrative review of meaning making and its effects on adjustment to stressful life events.' *Psychological Bulletin 136*(2), 257–301.

Peacock, S., Forbes, D., Markle-Reid, M., Hawranik, P. *et al.* (2010) 'The positive aspects of the caregiving journey with dementia: Using a strengths-based perspective to reveal opportunities.' *Journal of Applied Gerontology 29*(5), 640–659.

Pearlin, L.I. (1992) 'The careers of caregivers.' *The Gerontologist 32*, 647.

Pearlin, L.I., Mullan, J.T., Semple, S.J. and Skaff, M.M. (1990) 'Caregiving and the stress process: An overview of concepts and their measures.' *The Gerontologist 30*(5), 583–594.

Pinquart, M. and Sörensen, S. (2003) 'Differences between caregivers and noncaregivers in psychological health and physical health: A meta-analysis.' *Psychology and Aging 18*(2), 250–267.

Pruncho, R.A., Michaels, E. and Potashnik, S.L. (1990) 'Predictors of institutionalization among Alzheimer disease victims with caregiving spouses.' *Journals of Gerontology Social Sciences 45*(6), 259–266.

Quinn, C., Clare, L., McGuinness, T. and Woods, R.T. (2012) 'The impact of relationships, motivations, and meanings on dementia caregiving outcomes.' *International Psychogeriatrics 24*(11), 1816–1826.

Quinn, C., Clare, L. and Woods, R.T. (2010) 'The impact of motivations and meanings on the wellbeing of caregivers of people with dementia: A systematic review.' *International Psychogeriatrics 22*(1), 43–55.

Quinn, C., Clare, L. and Woods, R.T. (2012) 'What predicts whether caregivers of people with dementia find meaning in their role?' *International Journal of Geriatric Psychiatry 27*(11), 1195–1202.

Quinn, C., Clare, L. and Woods, R.T. (2015) 'Balancing needs: The role of motivations, meanings and relationship dynamics in the experience of informal caregivers of people with dementia.' *Dementia 14*(2), 220–237.

Rapp, S.R. and Chao, D. (2000) 'Appraisals of strain and of gain: Effects on psychological wellbeing of caregivers of dementia patients.' *Aging and Mental Health 4*(2), 142–147.

Saad, K., Hartman, J., Ballard, C., Kurian, M., Graham, C. and Wilcock, G. (1995) 'Coping by the carers of dementia sufferers.' *Age and Ageing 24*(6), 495–498.

Savundranayagam, M.Y. (2014) 'Receiving while giving: the differential roles of receiving help and satisfaction with help on caregiver rewards among spouses and adult-children.' *International Journal of Geriatric Psychiatry 29*(1), 41–48.

Semiatin, A.M. and O'Connor, M.K. (2012) 'The relationship between self-efficacy and positive aspects of caregiving in Alzheimer's disease caregivers.' *Aging and Mental Health 16*(6), 683–688.

Shim, B., Barroso, J., Gilliss, C.L. and Davis, L.L. (2013) 'Finding meaning in caring for a spouse with dementia.' *Applied Nursing Research 26*(3), 121–126.

Tennen, H. and Affleck, G. (2002) 'Benefit-finding and Benefit-reminding.' In C.R. Snyder and S.J. Lopez (eds) *Handbook of Positive Psychology.* New York, NY: Oxford University Press.

Zika, S. and Chamberlain, K. (1992) 'On the relation between meaning in life and psychological well-being.' *British Journal of Psychology 83*(1), 133–145.

Chapter 12

OVERVIEW AND WAYS FORWARD FOR A POSITIVE PSYCHOLOGY APPROACH TO DEMENTIA

Chris Clarke and Emma Wolverson, with
Charlotte Stoner and Aimee Spector

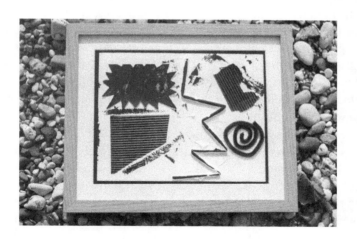

OVERVIEW

Positive psychology was deliberately (re)established as a separate field
because its pioneers were so disenchanted with an overriding focus
on pathology within mainstream psychology. Our research work in
dementia started from a similar place, with recognition of the continued

need to address an imbalance in dementia research, which has so far focused heavily on loss, deficit and decline. As clinicians and researchers in the field of dementia care, this did not match our experiences of how people live with dementia, nor does it match international health policy aspirations or the values and visions asserted by a growing dementia self-advocacy movement. The contents of this book not only highlight this paradox but also, we hope, show how a subjective lived experience perspective that is informed by a positive psychology approach helps re-balance the narratives that underpin our understanding of dementia.

This is not to say that important work to understand positive experiences in dementia has not already occurred or that we are proposing an entirely new field of study. Indeed, a key thread throughout this book has been the work of Kitwood (1997) and Sabat (2001), whose writings and research changed the way the experience of dementia is understood by placing the continued, active experience of well-being, identity and positive relationships in the foreground of people's lives. Furthermore, as this book has demonstrated, accounts of people living positively in spite of dementia have emerged within the lived experience literature, albeit often serendipitously. However, relatively little work has deliberately and systemically explored the strengths and resources of people living with dementia and how they experience positive well-being. A central message of this book is that positive experiences and attributes are fundamental aspects of personhood in dementia that should be explored directly and with the full collaboration of those living with the condition.

Surveying the varied chapters of this book highlights some key themes in relation to how well-being and living well in dementia might be further understood. First, we have seen how well-being reflects an interplay between positive and negative experiences, which can co-occur rather than simply displace each other. We have also seen how people actively strive towards using aspects of their personal and social 'capital' to maintain well-being as a vital part of their identity and personhood. At the same time, negative experiences in dementia (as in other adverse circumstances) could (re)activate forms of resilience or trigger a process of personal growth that can lead to positive outcomes for individuals. This is in line with second wave positive psychology perspectives (e.g. Lomas and Ivtzan, 2015) that draw attention to the interaction and interdependence between the positive and 'darker' sides of human experiences along the pathway to well-being and flourishing.

Second, the experience of dementia presents particular barriers to the utilisation of the positive strengths and resources that contribute to well-being. This may occur either directly due to cognitive impairment but, as many of the chapters suggest, this might be more likely to occur indirectly because of disabling social environments. The recognition that social contexts support and maintain well-being is, of course, not new in dementia care (Kitwood, 1993). What a positive psychology approach adds is a clearer account of the specific positive factors that social environments must facilitate in order to promote overall well-being. A positive psychology perspective also promotes a broader understanding of what helps communities to thrive, since no-one can live in a fulfilling or healthy way in a community at large that is 'sick'. A positive approach to the experience of well-being in dementia therefore needs to be fully contextualised, taking account of interactions between social, cultural, political and environmental factors (see Chapter 1). Such an approach is in keeping with social constructionist and relational approaches to selfhood in dementia (e.g. Sabat, 2001), moving beyond individualised, intra-personal accounts of well-being that have prevailed in positive psychology (Christopher and Hickinbottom, 2008). Importantly, by balancing individualist and collectivist perspectives, it will be possible to seek positive outcomes for individuals living with dementia as well as the inter-dependent social networks that surround and support them (Wong, 2011; see also Chapter 10).

Third, we have seen the recurring theme of how positive factors, resources, and well-being in dementia intersect with experiences of life-span development and ageing. People live with dementia in the context not only of their life-history but also of their life-stage, and this includes subjective experiences of ageing successfully as well as the motivation to experience positive emotion, achieve wisdom and seek transcendence. As such, people might not always place dementia in the foreground of their subjective experiences as they age and seek to maintain positive well-being.

CAUTIONS

As we have seen across several chapters, the risk of 'mandating' positive experiences and of not fully recognising the potential value of negative emotions and experience in fostering positive change is very relevant to exploring positive well-being in dementia, where there can already be a tendency to de-contextualise and de-personalise lived experiences on a social level. As we seek to further the application of positive psychology to dementia, we echo again that our intention is in no way to make light of the experience of dementia. We must be cautious about extrapolating individual positive experiences to understanding well-being on a group level; we can by no means assume that experiences of hope, humour or creativity, as examples, are accessible to all or are possible all of the time. We do not yet know how flourishing is best understood and measured in the context of living with dementia.

Moving beyond an artificial and arbitrary division between positive and negative experiences or processes is a necessary part of avoiding any kind of 'tyranny' being associated with a positive perspective on dementia. As noted, a dialectical positive psychology approach is highly relevant here; it helps reduce the risk of invalidating people's experiences because they are seen in a holistic and contextualised way. Positive psychology is not intended to replace what is known about suffering or disorder but to supplement it, and this is highly pertinent to dementia: 'No one should be criticized for not finding positive aspects of this disease [Alzheimer's disease], but no one should be overlooked who has found gifts amid such loss' (Stucky et al., 2002, p.206).

Many of the accounts and discussions presented within this book derive from small-scale qualitative studies, often based on humanistic and person-centred principles rather than the quantitative and nomothetic approach to research traditionally associated with positive psychology. On the one hand, this is a deliberately open and curious approach to fostering new theory where little is currently known and where loss-deficit and 'othering' discourses have tended to prevail. Positive psychology itself has tended to neglect this kind of idiographic perspective, which can potentially reveal much about what influences well-being across time and situations (Ong and Zautra, 2009).

On the other hand, a key limitation of the idiographic approach, and of the current literature base, is that it is difficult to systematically comprehend, organise and integrate islands of knowledge about positive experiences with each other and with mainstream thought and practice in dementia. At this stage, we also have to be very cautious about generalising the findings of such research to people living with various forms and severities of dementia – existing work has tended to focus on people living with early-stage dementia in developed nations, for instance. Moving forward, what is needed is an integration of qualitative and quantitative methods, at both individual and group levels, so that optimal experiences and well-being in different forms and severities of dementia, occurring in varying social contexts, can be fully understood.

TOWARDS A FRAMEWORK FOR THE APPLICATION OF POSITIVE PSYCHOLOGY TO DEMENTIA

In Chapter 2 we outlined the beginnings of a positive, person-centred approach to understanding living well with dementia by highlighting key connections between person-centred factors and corresponding positive psychology constructs. This enabled us to propose specific implications for living well with dementia (i.e. potential positive outcomes) as well as how social environments need to facilitate this. Given that the literature in this area is relatively nascent, this was necessarily tentative and remains so. However, we propose that this straightforward taxonomy holds value as an early attempt to link the potential theory of a positive person-centred approach with the practice of living well.

In light of all that has been presented and discussed in the preceding chapters, perhaps now we can also consider how the further development of a conceptual framework for the application of positive psychology to understanding lived experiences and well-being in dementia might proceed. A conceptually strong framework, based on the application of positive psychology, would provide a useful 'counter-frame' (Van Gorp and Vercruysse, 2012) to loss-deficit and biomedical narratives. This should spur further research into positive experiences, processes and outcomes in dementia and enable this research to form and be seen as a coherent whole, rather than as a collection of anomalous exceptions. This endeavour should eventually inform the development of therapeutic and community-based interventions or programmes aimed at maximising well-being in dementia.

Admittedly, these are lofty ambitions. We still have much to learn about which positive constructs or processes are most meaningful and influential for the well-being of people living with dementia. Concepts such as gratitude, self-compassion and love in dementia (as well as many more) await formal investigation. In addition, work is only beginning to outline what kinds of positive outcomes are most important for people with dementia as well as how these should best be measured, as discussed below. The premature development of a theoretical model could constrain or bias the scope of future research and, ironically, therefore prevent further important questions from being asked.

Perhaps all that should be attempted at this stage is to outline ways in which it might be possible to move towards developing useful frameworks for the application of positive psychology to dementia.

AN OVERARCHING, PROCESS-BASED ACCOUNT

At a meta-theoretical level, the themes and accounts presented in this book suggest how positive outcomes in experiences of dementia (i.e. living well) might result from interactions between:

- positive characteristics of the person (e.g. character strengths and virtues developed across the life-span and sustained in dementia)

- positive aspects of the social environment (accepting and mutually supportive relationships and networks where there is also positive well-being)

- positive psycho-social processes (see Du Plessis, 2014; e.g. maintaining hopefulness; fostering resilience; experiencing flow through creative activity).

Age-related developments, changes and challenges in dementia could, in theory, 'wrap around' these interacting factors and moderate relationships between them as people experience dementia over time. For example, positive development over the life-span could confer character strengths and virtues that foster personal growth, which in turn promotes aspects of flourishing in dementia (e.g. engagement, meaning and positive relationships). Alternatively, the experience of stigma and lowered personal agency in the context of progressive cognitive impairments could reduce the potential for positive processes to be fostered and sustained or contribute to positive outcomes in living with dementia. At different times, age-related developmental goals and concerns could be in the foreground of people's experiences, with challenges and changes relating to dementia in the background, and vice versa.

This potential framework, illustrated in Figure 12.1, represents a tentative proposal. It may not prove feasible to construct a 'grand theory' of positive psychology in relation to dementia, given the myriad individual differences in possible pathways to well-being and the multi-layered impact of the social environment. Furthermore, as we have seen throughout the chapters of this book, there may not be neat divisions between these meta-level categories in practice. Hope, for example, can be conceptualised simultaneously as a personal strength, a positive personal process and a positive relational factor. Similarly, resilience might be framed as a characteristic of the individual, an aspect of the social environment and as a measurable positive outcome. Further work is needed to identify how positive factors inter-relate in dementia and to what extent they act as mediators of the experience of well-being in dementia or as outcomes in their own right.

Importantly, any useful conceptual framework for the application of positive psychology principles to dementia should incorporate a dialectical perspective where well-being can be understood in terms of an interplay or between opposing forces or factors in people's everyday lives. There may be various levels at which this occurs. As indicated, well-being in dementia could involve achieving the right balance between challenges and resources (as well as positive and negative states) that still allows for an overall positive sense of self, relationships and personal meanings. A tension between positive ageing and confronting or responding to the changes and challenges that dementia can bring, as has been discussed, may be another level at which people living with dementia seek a positive balance. Similarly, other work has highlighted how adjusting to living with dementia can involve 'oscillating' between maintaining one's sense of self and adjusting self-concept to accommodate dementia's presence and impact (e.g. Clare, 2002).

Life-span development and ageing

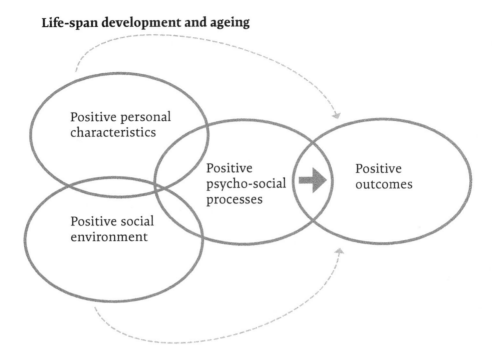

Dementia-related challenges and changes

*Figure 12.1: Possible framework for understanding
positive processes and outcomes in dementia*

POSITIVE DOMAINS OF FUNCTIONING IN DEMENTIA

The potential relevance of Rusk and Waters' (2014) empirical model of positive functioning to living positively with dementia was outlined in Chapter 2. This systems-based model focuses on observable and potentially measurable positive behaviours and characteristics, similar to the framework of indicators of relative well-being underpinning Dementia Care Mapping or the Bradford Well-Being Profile (Bradford Dementia Group, 2008). This makes it relevant to developing and refining positive interventions that could enhance specific aspects of psycho-social functioning, in order to produce positive outcomes for people living with dementia. In dementia, this is important since if certain domains of positive functioning become restricted (whether because of dementia directly or due to impoverished social environments) it may still be possible to nurture and enhance others to improve well-being.

Adapting this model to understanding living well in dementia would require further empirical work. We do not yet know whether domains of positive functioning (and relationships between them) differ in dementia. Notwithstanding this, we might be able to venture some initial ideas about the possible content of each domain in relation to living with dementia, based on the topics, themes and subjective accounts presented in this book and beyond (see 'Domains' below).

POTENTIAL 'DOMAINS' OF POSITIVE FUNCTIONING IN DEMENTIA (BASED ON RUSK AND WATERS, 2014)

ATTENTION AND AWARENESS

- attention towards present moment experiences
- awareness of maintained strengths and abilities
- experiences of flow through immersion in creative and meaningful activities.

COMPREHENSION AND COPING

- coping based on acceptance and meaning making
- retaining hopefulness grounded in reality
- cognitive re-appraisal; benefit finding
- showing resilience
- experiencing personal growth.

EMOTIONS

- expressing and appreciating humour
- experiencing and expressing love
- openness to joy, awe, gratitude and other positive emotions.

GOALS AND HABITS

- perseverance and courage
- engagement in meaningful and creative activities
- agency; self-determined choices and actions that are personally meaningful.

VIRTUES AND RELATIONSHIPS

- engaging reciprocally in positive, loving relationships
- volunteerism and activism
- intimacy and couplehood
- maintaining spirituality.

. . . .

DEFINING AND MEASURING WELL-BEING IN DEMENTIA – SHIFTING AWARENESS

The quantitative and nomothetic methods typically preferred within positive psychology frequently involve the use of outcome measurement. Outcome measurements usually take the form of questionnaires that aim to assess the degree to which a construct, issue or problem in question is present for a person, in a quantitative format. Examples of measures rooted in positive psychology within other domains are numerous. For example: the Herth Hope Index (Herth, 1992), developed for use in clinical settings; the Control, Autonomy, Self-Realisation and Pleasure (CASP-19; see Hyde *et al.*, 2003), developed for older adults; the Brief Resilience Scale (Smith, *et al.*, 2008), developed for those with a chronic illness; and the Care-Receiver Self-Efficacy Scale, for those with functional disabilities (Cox *et al.*, 2006).

Previously, outcome measures in dementia have been developed from a rather more negative viewpoint. Examples include attempting to relieve depression, anxiety or neuropsychiatric symptoms with the overarching goal of improving or maintaining 'cognition'. Even recent research appears to be preoccupied with the reduction of such states and thereby appears to infer well-being by the reduction or absence of these states (e.g. see Whitaker, *et al.*, 2014). Furthermore, clinicians and researchers have questioned the ability of a person with dementia to make a coherent and accurate self-judgement as cognition declines, and, as such, proxy raters (often carers) are often used to complete outcome measures on a participant's behalf.

Indeed, it is only recently that people with dementia themselves have been asked to give a view. This may be partly attributable to an emerging awareness of the variance between answers given by proxies and people with dementia (Burke, *et al.*, 1998; Gilley, *et al.*, 1995; Ott and Fogel, 1992) and the emergence of the person-centred care framework, in which the importance of the person's subjective views was first proposed (Kitwood, 1997). A shift in attitudes towards outcome measurement for people with dementia is most clearly illustrated by work conducted on Cognitive Stimulation Therapy (CST) trials. As the research was being developed, proxy raters were used to assess its efficacy. However, more recent trials favour ratings on measures from the participants themselves (Spector, *et al.*, 2003; Yates *et al.*, 2015). Again, the prevailing myth of people with dementia being unable to engage in outcome evaluation is debunked when we look at other domains specific to dementia, where self-report outcome measures have been successfully developed to assess physical functioning (Bucks *et al.*, 1996) and quality of life (Logsdon *et al.*, 1999). For people familiar with Kitwood's work, this will be common sense. However, previous conceptualisations of positive well-being in dementia could be accused of misconstruing positive attributes as a means of denial or reducing them down to a coping mechanism that is employed to manage losses and deficits incurred (Macquarrie, 2005).

'QUALITY OF LIFE'

Quality of life has now long been seen as a desirable outcome within psycho-social dementia research, and this concept can be related to positive psychology principles in certain ways (see Chapter 3). Although it has been suggested that below a certain level of cognitive function it is difficult to appraise one's quality of life, some people still appear able to give a view, even with severe impairment (Moyle *et al.*, 2011).

It is suggested that the shift to measuring 'quality of life' is the first step in a long process of recognising the positive states and emotions that people with dementia experience and measuring such positive states in a scientifically robust manner. Whilst quality of life research has contributed to a wealth of understanding, it is a term that is abstract in nature and tends to lack a theoretical basis. A focus on more clearly defined positive outcomes (e.g. PERMA (see Chapter 1); Seligman, 2011) and particular kinds of well-being (e.g. hedonic versus eudemonic) could contribute to the development of measures that are conceptually strong as well as valid.

CURRENT USES OF POSITIVE PSYCHOLOGY MEASURES

Positive psychology outcome measures are beginning to be adopted for use in psycho-social intervention research for people with dementia. Examples include the Rosenberg Self-Esteem scale (Rosenberg, 1965) and the General Self-Efficacy scale (Schwarzer and Jerusalem, 1995) utilised in a healthy behaviours promotion trial (Buettner and Fitzsimmons, 2009). However, researchers appear to be picking such measures off the shelf, often without reporting a rationale or examining the scale's psychometric properties for people with dementia. Unsurprisingly, results from such studies have been varied. As such, currently there are so few studies within positive psychology and dementia that a definitive statement upon the efficacy of measuring such positive attributes cannot be made at present.

POTENTIAL WAYS FORWARD

To date, no positive psychology measures have been developed within the various domains of this discipline specifically for people with dementia. A lack of gold standard outcome measures means that positive psychology is in its infancy with regard to the measurement of positive attributes, experiences and outcomes for them. The qualitative literature provides a strong rationale for the development of robust outcome measures to further investigate aspects of positive well-being for people with dementia. Developing such measures specifically for people with dementia would allow positive characteristics to be defined in the way that is most valid and suitable for this population. These may or may not be identical to other populations, but until it is properly investigated it cannot be assumed one way or another. In order to make this a reality, people with dementia must be included at every stage of the development procedure to ensure that appropriate measures for this population are developed. A means of accomplishing this may be facilitating focus groups of people with dementia to collaboratively produce conceptualisations of positive concepts or aspects of well-being as they relate to their own lived experiences and to generate items verbatim for the design of new measures. This would ensure that developed measures have high levels of content validity for this population (see Mountain, Moniz-Cook and Øksnebjerg, 2015, for a more detailed discussion of how new psycho-social outcome measures in dementia may be developed).

Whilst such measures are being developed, researchers could potentially examine scales that have been successfully used in populations that have shared characteristics to those of dementia. A recent review identified such measures for populations of chronic illness, traumatic brain injury and older adults. The authors of this review undertook a detailed quality assessment of these measures and made appropriate recommendations for which scales could be adapted for people with dementia in areas of resilience, self-efficacy, religiousness/spirituality, life valuation, autonomy, sense of coherence and resourcefulness (Stoner, Orrell and Spector, 2015). These measures, as well as more general positive psychology outcome measures that could be relevant to the measurement of well-being in dementia are shown in Table 12.1.

In summary, qualitative research conducted to date provides a clear rationale for the development of scientifically robust outcome measures that can assess positive constructs identified as present and meaningful for people with dementia. This will allow for an in-depth investigation of the role of positive psychology within dementia in a quantifiable manner. The scientific study of such constructs may lead to important advances in the field, including more targeted psycho-social interventions and less preoccupation with the measurement of 'static' health-related quality of life at one time point (see Mountain, Moniz-Cook and Øksnebjerg, 2015).

Table 12.1: Measures of positive outcomes potentially relevant to dementia

DOMAIN	OUTCOME MEASURE	BRIEF DESCRIPTION	POPULATION/GROUPS DEVELOPED AND USED WITH	APPLICATION TO DEMENTIA
Flourishing	Flourishing Scale (Diener *et al.*, 2010)	8 items covering social relationships, purpose and meaning in life, engagement, self-respect, optimism, competence and capability. 7-point Likert scale with responses ranging from '1 – strongly disagree' to '7 – strongly agree'. Higher scores reflect higher degree of flourishing	1) University students (n=689; male=175, female=468) 2) Portuguese full-time employees and undergraduate students (n=911): internal consistency high and acceptable correlation with life satisfaction (Junça Silva and Caetano, 2013)	A potential self-report measure of aspects of positive psychological well-being, including purpose, meaning, self-esteem, hope/optimism as well as reciprocity and support in social relationships.
Positive and negative affect	Scale of Positive and Negative Experience (SPANE) (Diener *et al.*, 2010)	12-item, 5-point Likert scale with responses ranging from '1 – very rarely or never' to '5 – very often or always'. Higher scores reflect higher degree of positive affect	1) University students (n=689; male=175, female=468) 2) Portuguese full-time employees and undergraduate students (n=911): internal consistency high and acceptable correlation with life satisfaction (Junça Silva and Caetano, 2013)	A potential self-report measure of the balance between positive and negative emotional experiences, from the perspective of the person. These may occur over time or in the moment.

Resilience	Connor–Davidson Resilience Scale (Connor and Davidson, 2003)	25-item scale, 5-point Likert scale (0–4), with responses ranging from '0 – not true at all' to '4 – nearly all the time'. Higher scores reflect greater resilience	1) American sample (n=806; mean age 43.8) 2) General population (non-help-seeking) 3) Primary care recipients 4) Psychiatric outpatients 5) Generalised anxiety disorder (GAD) and Post traumatic stress disorder (PTSD) 6) Older adults (age range 55–75+): excellent internal consistency (Goins, Gregg and Fiske, 2013)	A self-assessed measure of the presence of personal resilience.
Spirituality	Geriatric Spiritual Wellbeing Scale (Dunn, 2008)	16-item scale covering affirmative self-appraisal, connectedness, altruistic benevolence and faith pathways. 6-point Likert scale with responses ranging from '1 – strongly disagree' to '6 – strongly agree'	American community dwelling older adults (n=138; mean age 74.2). Good internal consistency and test–retest reliability	A potential measure of well-being based on spiritual principles. Domains include: affirmation of life, feeling connected to others and religious faith.
Autonomy	Maastricht Personal Autonomy Questionnaire (MPAQ) (Mars et al, 2014)	16 items covering degree of autonomy and working on autonomy. 5-point Likert scale. Three sub-scales: 'living the way you want; arranging your life; doing what you enjoy and doing what's best for your health'	Older adults with chronic physical illness (see Mars et al, 2014).	A measure of personal autonomy for older adults with a chronic illness.

DOMAIN	OUTCOME MEASURE	BRIEF DESCRIPTION	POPULATION/GROUPS DEVELOPED AND USED WITH	APPLICATION TO DEMENTIA
Sense of coherence	Sense of Coherence Scale (Antonovsky, 1993)	29-item or 13-item short form (SF), 7-point semantic differential scale	Validation study of 13 items in Dutch young adults with chronic illness: (n=2781) 14–18- and 19–25-year-olds scored lowest, whereas 14–18-year-olds with congenital heart disease and 26–30-year-olds scored highest, irrespective of gender. A confirmatory factor analysis (CFA) resulted in items 5 and 6 being dropped. 3 sub-scales of meaningfulness, comprehensibility and manageability loaded onto a single second-order factor (Luyckx et al., 2012)	A measure consisting of three components: comprehensibility, manageability and meaningfulness.
Resourcefulness	The Resourcefulness Scale for Older Adults (RSOA) (Zauszniewski, Lai and Tithiphontumrong, 2006)	28-item, 6-point Likert scale. 2 sub-scales: personal resourcefulness and social resourcefulness	Older adults (n=451; mean age: 81). Average of 3 chronic health conditions per participant	A measure of perceived ability to independently perform daily tasks (personal resourcefulness), and to seek help from others when unable to function independently (social resourcefulness).
Motivation	Control, Autonomy, Self-Realisation and Pleasure (CASP-19) (Hyde et al., 2003)	19-item self-report scale, 4-point Likert scale. Responses ranged from '0 – never' to '3 – often'	Older adults with chronic physical illness (n=412; mean age: 70.25)	A second order measure, which views quality of life as the satisfaction of four domains: Control, Autonomy, Self-realisation and Pleasure.

Example item:
'I look forward to each day.' |

| Life valuation | The Satisfaction with Life Scale (SWLS) (Diener et al, 1985) | 5-item self-report scale, 7-point Likert scale. Responses range from '1 – strongly disagree' to '7 – strongly agree'. Includes a neutral mid-point 4 – neither agree nor disagree' | 1) American undergraduate students at University of Illinois (sample 1: n=176; sample 2: n=176) 2) Validation in Turkish older adults (n=123). Convergent validity: positively correlated with self-esteem, perceived current health status whilst negatively correlated with depression (Durak, Senol-Durak and Gencoz, 2010) 3) Spanish translation and analysis (n=266). Analysis of factorial variance between adolescents (n=133) and older adults (n=133). Acceptable 1-factor model for both adolescents and older adults found (Pons et al., 2000) 4) Portuguese translation and validation in older adults (n=1003): internal consistency high. Convergent validity: positively correlated with perceived health and generativity (Sancho et al., 2014) | A measure of self-perceived satisfaction with life (an aspect of subjective well-being) rather than illness-related quality of life. |

SOME IMPLICATIONS FOR CLINICAL PRACTICE IN DEMENTIA

As Phinney highlighted in Chapter 3, whilst attempting to present themselves as an alternative to medical treatments, psycho-social interventions in dementia have actually tended to follow a medicalised approach, focusing on the amelioration of negative states and experiences that are often framed as 'symptoms' of dementia (e.g. see Livingston *et al.*, 2005). If we see positive well-being as a process that does not merely equate to the absence of negative emotions, dysfunctional thoughts or maladaptive behaviours (Keyes, 2005), then psycho-social interventions in dementia should instead focus on how to best support people to maximise their personal and social strengths and assets.

Accordingly, as Phinney outlines, existing interventions and approaches might be used more effectively if they are directly aimed at enhancing the *presence* of positive processes likely to underpin subjective and psychological well-being in dementia. Life-story and reminiscence work, for instance, may boost positive well-being (over time or in the moment) insofar as it strengthens personal meaning, hope and reciprocal social interactions (see Wu and Koo, 2015). Physical exercise could specifically promote the experience of positive emotion through the enhancement of self-determination and flow. There is, potentially, a long list of other interventions whose aims could be similarly framed in terms of aspects of flourishing, subjective well-being or resilience. However, previous research into the effectiveness of such interventions has not tended to consider their impact on these positive outcomes or which particular positive psycho-social processes they might operate on to produce them. This is an important avenue for continued research.

As we learn more about the factors (or domains of functioning) most pertinent to positive well-being in dementia, there is the potential to develop new interventions or programmes to specifically target these. This could involve the adaptation of existing positive interventions such as humour therapies (Low *et al.*, 2013), hope therapy (e.g. Cheavens *et al.*, 2006), or resilience-focused cognitive-behaviour therapy (e.g. Padesky and Mooney, 2012). These might be seen as 'stand-alone' interventions and may differ in how acceptable and effective they are in achieving positive outcomes for different people living with dementia. A more fruitful approach could be to develop positive intervention programmes that target a range of interconnected positive processes that are most relevant to well-being in dementia. An analogous programme can be found in the work of Ramirez and colleagues (2013) who developed a multi-component positive intervention based on the integration of gerontological concepts and positive psychology. This specifically targeted the enhancement of positive autobiographical memories in conjunction with the fostering of forgiveness and gratitude with respect to life-span issues. Amongst 46 older people (aged 60–93), the group-based intervention was shown to have significant effects on positive outcomes in particular, namely increasing levels of life satisfaction and subjective well-being.

An alternative approach will be to develop individually tailored approaches, rather than standardised group interventions, to target both positive psychological processes and outcomes in dementia. The potential for individual differences to occur in the extent to which different positive activities impact on well-being has been of interest to positive psychology researchers (see Lyubomirsky and Layous, 2013) and is an important consideration in relation to dementia. In a key illustration of this, Van Haistma and colleagues (2015) conducted a randomised controlled trial to test the effectiveness of individualised activity programmes for 180 nursing home residents living with dementia. The design of these bespoke programmes was underpinned by self-determination theory (aiming to meet needs for autonomy, connectedness and competence) and the broaden-and-build theory of positive emotion (Fredrickson, 2004). Residents receiving this intervention showed significant improvements in positive emotion and positive verbal behaviour, as compared with standardised one-to-one activities or care as usual. Not only do such findings demonstrate how positive psychology constructs are applicable to improving well-being in dementia, they also illustrate how positive outcomes are more likely to be achieved when a 'fit' occurs between positive activities being undertaken and the strengths and resources of the person.

Receiving a diagnosis is one of the most critical points in the dementia 'journey' in relation to the subsequent experience of well-being (see Aminzadeh et al., 2007). Because a truly positive approach is proactive rather than reactive to the emergence of negative experiences, it is here that health professionals have a key early opportunity to work with people and their families to explore how they can maintain and build their well-being in living with dementia. Diagnostic disclosure should not be treated as a task separate to this process (see Moniz-Cook and Manthorpe, 2008). Actively promoting well-being as part of diagnostic disclosure is, in some nations, already a best practice approach (e.g. see Hodge, Hailey and Orrell, 2014), but it is not clear whether health professionals, in practice, always feel able to convey hope, promote agency and foster narratives based around aspects of well-being such as meaning and engagement (Vince, Clarke and Wolverson, 2015). This might be because of a perceived lack of post-diagnosis support services available or a more general sense of hopelessness around dementia that reflects the dominance of a loss-deficit narrative (see Moore and Cahill, 2013). An approach to diagnostic disclosure and post-diagnostic support that is focused on fostering the subjective experience of resilience could be a key way forward here. As Harris (Chapter 6) suggests, this would direct health professionals towards facilitating acceptance and meaning-based positive coping, hope, engagement in activity and reciprocally rewarding social relationships. Training programmes for health and social care professionals that incorporate resilience and how it can be identified and maintained in dementia are essential to embed this approach in practice.

In its focus on subjective well-being and the uniqueness of the individual, person-centred care should intuitively focus on how aspects of well-being are experienced and expressed by each individual. What a positive psychology approach potentially adds is an emphasis on maximising the optimal positive well-being of the person with dementia, as far beyond the 'baseline' as is possible. Dementia care environments need to be designed and staffed on the basis of this overarching aim. A positive approach also offers a deeper understanding of the dimensions and domains of well-being and how they can be enhanced. Three particular implications for dementia care can be delineated:

1. People bring positive personal strengths to living with dementia as aspects of selfhood. These may or may not be changed by dementia, and good care should involve identifying them and creating conditions and relationships that maintain and nurture their use.

2. A deliberate focus on maintaining personal strengths and creating conditions that are conducive to having optimal experiences adds a further dimension to the 'positive person work' required to maintain personhood and well-being in

dementia (Kitwood, 1997). As such, carers are seeking to promote experiences of pleasure, joy, hope, humour, engagement, flow, playfulness, agency, reciprocity and even transcendence, depending on a balance between the strengths and needs of the person with dementia and the positive challenges that can be provided by a supportive social environment.

3. As Nolan and Ryan (Chapter 10), highlight, levels of well-being in the social environment are likely to impact on that of the person with dementia. Literature elsewhere supports this notion; subjective well-being and life satisfaction 'spread' through social networks, even where relationships are indirect (Fowler and Christakis, 2008). In dementia care, a key implication is that promoting subjective and psychological well-being amongst carers and members of the social network is likely to enhance care and foster increased well-being for people who have dementia.

IMPLICATIONS FOR PUBLIC POLICY– MOVING THE DEMENTIA DISCOURSE FORWARD

From a public health perspective, improving average levels of well-being (i.e. increasing the numbers of people in the population who are 'flourishing' rather than 'languishing'; see Huppert, 2009) by even a small degree has a powerful effect on individual levels of well-being. This is highly pertinent to dementia. Given its individual, social and societal impact and attendant risks of psychological and physical morbidity, it is now recognised as a world-wide public health priority (World Health Organization, 2012). As such, raising well-being in dementia on a population level is now a priority for us all. However, we have yet to establish the prevalence of subjective or psychological well-being in the population of people living with dementia. A baseline is needed to inform and drive improvements in well-being in dementia at the population level that are based on building strengths and resources pre- and post-diagnosis, not just preventing morbidity and burden. These will be important ways to address dementia as a public health issue.

A key vehicle for addressing well-being at this level also lies in the design and implementation of effective health policies. Whilst, in recent years, dementia-related health policies in many countries have pursued a 'living well' message, this has been somewhat ambiguous and not informed, as yet, by a positive psychological perspective on well-being. As Innes and Manthorpe (2013) argue, the way that dementia is framed and conceptualised will influence how policy initiatives are formed and implemented. Whilst the notion of living well was enshrined in England's pioneering National Dementia Strategy (Department of Health, 2009), in practice it was primarily framed in relation to improving healthcare systems around the person and was therefore implicitly based on a biomedical perspective. As Innes and Manthorpe (2013) highlight, social-psychological and gerontological perspectives on dementia could enrich health policies towards improving the lived experiences of individuals and improving social discourses that surround the condition.

We suggest that a positive psychology approach further complements both of these perspectives in several ways. First, it will help specify what is really meant by living well (i.e. linking it to positive psycho-social processes and relevant well-being outcomes) and the different pathways by which this might be achieved. A positive, theory-based approach could also help ensure that health policy interventions are well-being- and asset-focused, promoting individualised, positive care approaches as well as the well-being and 'capital' of social networks around the person with dementia. A potentially powerful policy intervention will be to frame subjective and psychological well-being in dementia as a public health outcome against which organisations and services could be evaluated.

Health policies based on a positive bio-psycho-social conceptualisation of dementia have further potential in promoting positive images and narratives that raise expectations and further reducing the 'othering' of people living with the condition. A challenge for future policy makers will be how to prioritise dementia as a public health concern whilst implementing policies that address personal and social well-being and promote messages and images of living well. To avoid any 'mandating' of positivity at a social/political level, a dialectical positive psychology approach could help create a balanced perspective on well-being in dementia. This could help instil more hopeful and compassionate narratives about what living well with the condition can actually mean, potentially increasing people's readiness to access services and seek a diagnosis in an autonomous and timely way. Overall, policy initiatives based on these concepts could assist 'dementia-friendly' communities to go one step further to become 'dementia-positive', geared not only towards accepting dementia and supporting inclusion but also actively promoting and improving positive well-being.

Having the opportunity to flourish whilst living with dementia need not be a utopian dream. This book represents a step towards understanding how it can be made an individual reality. Positive health policies that drive dementia-positive communities, services and research towards fostering positive lived-experiences in dementia are worthy and achievable aspirations that are increasingly relevant to us all.

REFERENCES

Aminzadeh, F., Byszewski, A., Molnar, F.J. and Eisner, M. (2007) 'Emotional impact of dementia diagnosis: Exploring persons with dementia and caregivers' perspectives.' *Aging and Mental Health 11*(3), 281–290.

Antonovsky, A. (1993) 'The structure and properties of the sense of coherence scale.' *Social Science and Medicine 36*, 725–733.

Bucks, R.S., Ashworth, D.L., Wilcock, G.K. and Siegfried, K. (1996) 'Assessment of activities of daily living in dementia: Development of the Bristol Activities of Daily Living Scale.' *Age and Ageing 25*, 113–120.

Buettner, L.L. and Fitzsimmons, S. (2009) 'Promoting health in early-stage dementia: Evaluation of a 12-week course.' *Journal of Gerontological Nursing 35*(3), 39–49.

Bradford Dementia Group (2008) *The Bradford Well-Being Profile*. University of Bradford. Available at www.bradford.ac.uk/health/media/healthmedia/Bradford-Well-Being-Profile-with-cover-(3).pdf, accessed on 12 May 2016.

Burke, W.J., Roccaforte, W.H., Wengel, S.P., McArthur-Miller, D., Folks, D.G. and Potter, J.F. (1998) 'Disagreement in the reporting of depressive symptoms between patients with dementia of the Alzheimer type and their collateral sources.' *American Journal of Geriatric Psychiatry 6*, 308–319.

Cheavens, J.S., Feldman, D.B., Gum, A., Michael, S.T. and Snyder, C.R. (2006) 'Hope therapy in a community sample: A pilot investigation.' *Social Indicators Research 77*(1), 61–78.

Christopher, J.C. and Hickinbottom, S. (2008) 'Positive psychology, ethnocentrism, and the disguised ideology of individualism.' *Theory and Psychology 18*(5), 563–589.

Clare, L. (2002) 'We'll fight it as long as we can: Coping with the onset of Alzheimer's disease.' *Aging and Mental Health 6*, 139–148.

Connor, K.M. and Davidson, J.R. (2003) 'Development of a new resilience scale: The Connor–Davidson Resilience Scale (CD-RISC).' *Depression and Anxiety 18*, 76–82.

Cox, E.O., Green, K.E., Seo, H., Inaba, M. and Quillen, A.A (2006) 'Coping with late life challenges: Development and validation of the Care-Receiver Efficacy Scale.' *The Gerontologist 46*(5), 640–649.

Department of Health (2009) *Living Well With Dementia: A National Dementia Strategy.* London: Department of Health.

Diener, E., Emmons, R.A., Larsen, R.J. and Griffin, S. (1985) 'The satisfaction with life scale.' *Journal of Personality Assessment 49*(1), 71–75.

Diener, E., Wirtz, D., Tov, W., Kim-Prieto, C. *et al.*, (2010) 'New well-being measures: Short scales to assess flourishing and positive and negative feelings.' *Social Indicators Research 97*, 143–156.

Dunn, K.S. (2008) 'Development and psychometric testing of a new geriatric spiritual well-being scale.' *International Journal of Older People Nursing 3*, 161–169.

Du Plessis, G.A. (2014) *A meta-theoretical taxonomy of positive psychology constructs.* University of Johannesburg. Available at http://ujdigispace.uj.ac. za/bitstream/handle/10210/13527/Du%20Plessis%20G%20A%202014. pdf?sequence=1&isAllowed=y, accessed on 13 July 2016.

Durak, M., Senol-Durak, E. and Gencoz, T. (2010) 'Psychometric properties of the satisfaction with life scale among Turkish university students, correctional officers and elderly adults.' *Social Indicators Research 99*(3), 413–429.

Fredrickson, B.L. (2004) 'The broaden-and-build theory of positive emotions.' Philosophical Transactions of the Royal Society of London. *Series B: Biological Sciences 359*(1449), 1367–1377.

Gilley, D.W., Wilson, R.S., Fleischman, D.A., Harrison, D.W., Goetz, C.G. and Tanner, C.M. (1995) 'Impact of Alzheimer's-type dementia and information source on the assessment of depression.' *Psychological Assessment 7*, 42–48.

Goins, R.T., Gregg, J.J. and Fiske, A. (2013) 'Psychometric properties of the Connor–Davidson Resilience Scale with older American Indians: The native elder care study.' *Research on Aging 35*(2), 123–143.

Fowler, J.H. and Christakis, N.A. (2008) 'Dynamic spread of happiness in a large social network: Longitudinal analysis over 20 years in the Framingham Heart Study.' *British Medical Journal 337*, a2338.

Herth, K. (1992) 'Abbreviated instrument to measure hope: Development and psychometric evaluation.' *Journal of Advanced Nursing 17*, 1251–1259.

Hodge, S., Hailey, E. and Orrell, M. (2014) *Memory Services National Accreditation Programme (MSNAO): Standards for Memory Services.* Fourth edition. London: Royal College of Psychiatrists. Available at www.rcpsych.ac.uk/pdf/MSNAP%20 Standards%20Fourth%20Edition%202014r.pdf, accessed on 15 June 2016.

Huppert, F.A. (2009) 'Psychological well-being: Evidence regarding its causes and consequences.' *Applied Psychology: Health and Well-Being 1*(2), 137–164.

Hyde, M., Wiggins, R.D., Higgs, P. and Blane, D.B. (2003) 'A measure of quality of life in early old age: The theory, development and properties of a needs satisfaction model (CASP-19).' *Aging and Mental Health 7*(3), 186–194.

Innes, A. and Manthorpe, J. (2013) 'Developing theoretical understandings of dementia and their application to dementia care policy in the UK.' *Dementia 12*(6), 682–696.

Junça Silva, A. and Caetano, A. (2013) 'Validation of the flourishing scale and scale of positive and negative experience in Portugal.' *Social Indicators Research 110*, 469–478.

Keyes, C.L.M. and Lopez, S.J. (2005) 'Toward a Science of Mental Health.' In C.R Snyder and S.J. Lopez (eds) *Handbook of Positive Psychology*. New York, NY: Oxford University Press.

Kitwood, T. (1993) 'Towards a theory of dementia care: The interpersonal process.' *Ageing and Society 13*(1), 51–67.

Kitwood, T. (1997) *Dementia Reconsidered: The Person Comes First*. Buckingham: Open University Press.

Livingston, G., Johnston, K., Katona, C., Paton, J., Lyketsos, C.G., and Old Age Task Force of the World Federation of Biological Psychiatry. (2005) 'Systematic review of psychological approaches to the management of neuropsychiatric symptoms of dementia.' *American Journal of Psychiatry 162*(11), 1996–2021.

Logsdon, R.G., Gibbons, L.E., McCurry, S.M. and Teri, L. (1999) 'Quality of life in Alzheimer's disease: Patient and caregiver reports.' *Journal of Mental Health and Aging 5*, 21–32.

Lomas, T. and Ivtzan, I. (2015) 'Second wave positive psychology: Exploring the positive–negative dialectics of wellbeing.' *Journal of Happiness Studies*. DOI: http://dx.doi.org/10.1007/s10902-015-9668-y

Low, L.F., Brodaty, H., Goodenough, B., Spitzer, P. *et al.* (2013) 'The Sydney Multisite Intervention of LaughterBosses and ElderClowns (SMILE) study: Cluster randomised trial of humour therapy in nursing homes.' *BMJ Open 3*(1). DOI: 10.1136/bmjopen-2012-002072

Luyckx, K., Goossens, E., Apers, S., Rassart, J. *et al.* (2012) 'The 13-item sense of coherence scale in Dutch-speaking adolescents and young adults: Structural validity, age trends, and chronic disease.' *Psychologica Belgica 52*(4), 351–368.

Lyubomirsky, S. and Layous, K. (2013) 'How do simple positive activities increase wellbeing?' *Current Directions in Psychological Science 22*(1), 57–62.

Macquarrie, C.R. (2005) 'Experiences in early stage Alzheimer's disease: Understanding the paradox of acceptance and denial.' *Aging and Mental Health 9*(5), 430–441.

Mars, G.J., van Eijk, J.M., Post, M.W., Proot, I.M., Mesters, I. and Kempen, G.I. (2014) 'Development and psychometric properties of the Maastricht Personal Autonomy Questionnaire (MPAQ) in older adults with a chronic physical illness.' *Quality of Life Research 23*, 1777–1787.

Moniz-Cook, E. and Manthorpe, J. (eds) (2008) *Early Psychosocial Interventions in Dementia*. London: Jessica Kingsley Publishers.

Moore, V. and Cahill, S. (2013) 'Diagnosis and disclosure of dementia – A comparative qualitative study of Irish and Swedish General Practitioners.' *Aging and Mental Health 17*(1), 77–84.

Mountain, G., Moniz-Cook, E.D. and Øksnebjerg, L. (2015) *Dementia Outcome Measures: Charting New Territory* (Report of a JPND Working Group on Longitudinal Cohorts; EU Joint Programme Neurodegenerative Disease Research). Available at www.neurodegenerationresearch.eu/wp-content/uploads/2015/10/JPND-Report-Fountain.pdf, accessed on 23 April 2016.

Moyle, W., Gracia, N., Murfield, J.E., Griffiths, S.G. and Venturato, L. (2011) 'Assessing quality of life in older people with dementia in long-term care: A comparison of two self-report measures.' *Journal of Clinical Nursing 21*(11–12), 1632–1640.

Ong, A.D. and Zautra, A.J. (2009) 'Modeling Positive Human Health: From Covariance Structures to Dynamic Systems.' In C.R Snyder and S.J Lopez (eds) *Handbook of Positive Psychology*. New York, NY: Oxford University Press.

Ott, B. and Fogel, B.S. (1992) 'Measurement of depression in dementia: Self versus clinical rating.' *International Journal of Geriatric Psychiatry 7*, 899–904.

Padesky, C.A. and Mooney, K.A. (2012) 'Strengths-based cognitive–behavioural therapy: A four-step model to build resilience.' *Clinical Psychology and Psychotherapy 19*(4), 283–290.

Pons, D., Atienza, F.L., Balaguer, I. and Garcia-Merita, M.L. (2000) 'Satisfaction with life scale: Analysis of factorial invariance for adolescents and elderly persons.' *Perceptual and Motor Skills 91*(1), 62–68.

Ramirez, E., Ortega, A.R., Chamorro, A. and Colmenero, J.M. (2014) 'A program of positive intervention in the elderly: Memories, gratitude and forgiveness.' *Aging and Mental Health 18*(4), 463–470.

Rosenberg, M. (1965) *Society and the Adolescent Self-image*. Princeton, NJ: Princeton University Press.

Rusk, R.D. and Waters, L. (2014) 'A psycho-social system approach to well-being: Empirically deriving the Five Domains of Positive Functioning.' *The Journal of Positive Psychology 9*, 1–12.

Sabat, S.R. (2001) *The Experience of Alzheimer's Disease: Life Through a Tangled Veil*. Oxford: Blackwell.

Sancho, P., Galiana, L., Guiterrez, M., Francisco, E. and Tomas, J.M. (2014) 'Validating the Portugese version of the Satisfaction with Life Scale in an elderly sample.' *Social Indicators Research 115*(1), 457–466.

Schwarzer, R. and Jerusalem, M. (1995) 'Generalized Self-Efficacy Scale.' In J. Weinman, S. Wright and M. Johnston (eds) *Measures in Health Psychology: A User's Portfolio. Causal and Control Beliefs*. Windsor: NFER-Nelson.

Seligman, M.E.P. (2011) *Flourish: A Visionary New Understanding of Happiness and Well-being*. New York: NY: Simon & Schuster.

Smith, B.W., Dalen, J., Wiggins, K., Tooley, E., Christopher, P. and Bernard, J. (2008) 'The brief resilience scale: Assessing the ability to bounce back.' *International Journal of Behavioural Medicine 15*, 194–200.

Spector, A., Thorgrimsen, L., Woods, B., Royan, L., Davies, S., Butterworth, M. and Orrell, M. (2003) 'Efficact of an evidence-based cognitive stimulation therapy programme for people with dementia: Randomised controlled trial.' *British Journal of Psychiatry 183*, 248–254.

Stoner, C.R., Orrell, M. and Spector, A. (2015) 'Review of positive psychology outcome measures for chronic illness, traumatic brain injury and older adults: Adaptability in dementia.' *Dementia and Geriatric Cognitive Disorders 40*(5–6), 340–357.

Stucky, J.C., Post, S.G., Ollerton, S., FallCreek, S.J. and Whitehouse, P.J. (2002) 'Alzheimer's disease, religion and the ethics of respect for spirituality: A community dialogue.' *Alzheimer's Care Quarterly 3*(3), 199–207.

Van Gorp, B. and Vercruysse, T. (2012) 'Frames and counter-frames giving meaning to dementia: A framing analysis of media content.' *Social Science and Medicine 74*(8), 1274–1281.

Van Haitsma, K.S., Curyto, K., Abbott, K.M., Towsley, G.L., Spector, A. and Kleban, M. (2015) 'A randomized controlled trial for an individualized positive psychosocial intervention for the affective and behavioral symptoms of dementia in nursing home residents.' *Journal of Gerontology: Psychological and Social Sciences 70*(1), 35–45.

Vince, A., Clarke, C. and Wolverson, E.L. (2015) *An exploration of psychiatrists' experiences of discussing living well and positive wellbeing when sharing a diagnosis of dementia* (unpublished manuscript). University of Hull.

Whitaker, R., Fossey, J., Ballard, C., Orrell, M. *et al.* (2014) 'Improving well-being and health for people with dementia (WHELD): Study protocol for a randomised controlled trial.' *Trials.* DOI: 10.1186/1745-6215-15-284

Wong, P.T.P. (2011) 'Positive psychology 2.0: Towards a balanced interactive model of the good life.' *Canadian Psychology 52*(2), 69–81.

World Health Organization (WHO) (2012) *Dementia: A Public Health Priority.* World Health Organization.

Wu, L.F., and Koo, M. (2015) 'Randomized controlled trial of a six-week spiritual reminiscence intervention on hope, life satisfaction, and spiritual well-being in elderly with mild and moderate dementia.' *International Journal of Geriatric Psychiatry 31*(2), 120–127.

Yates, L.A., Orrell, M., Spector, A. and Orgeta, V. (2015) 'Service users' involvement in the development of individual Cognitive Stimulation Therapy (iCST) for dementia: A qualitative study.' *BioMed Central Geriatrics 15*(4), 1–10.

Zauszniewski, J.A., Lai, C. and Tithiphontumrong, S. (2006) Development and testing of the resourcefulness scale for older adults.' *Journal of Nursing Management 14*(1), 57–68.

SUBJECT INDEX

AUTHOR INDEX